ORTHOPEDIC CLINICS OF NORTH AMERICA

www.orthopedic.theclinics.com

Surgical Considerations for Osteoporosis, Osteopenia, and Vitamin D Deficiency

April 2019 • Volume 50 • Number 2

ELSEVIER

1600 John F. Kennedy Boulevard • Suite 1800 • Philadelphia, Pennsylvania, 19103-2899.

http://www.orthopedic.theclinics.com

ORTHOPEDIC CLINICS OF NORTH AMERICA Volume 50, Number 2
April 2019 ISSN 0030-5898, ISBN-13: 978-0-323-65513-2

Editor: Lauren Boyle
Developmental Editor: Kristen Helm

Photocopying

Single photocopies of single articles may be made for personal use as allowed by national copyright laws. Permission of the Publisher and payment of a fee is required for all other photocopying, including multiple or systematic copying, copying for advertising or promotional purposes, resale, and all forms of document delivery. Special rates are available for educational institutions that wish to make photocopies for non-profit educational classroom use. For information on how to seek permission visit www.elsevier.com/permissions or call: (+44) 1865 843830 (UK)/(+1) 215 239 3804 (USA).

Derivative Works

Subscribers may reproduce tables of contents or prepare lists of articles including abstracts for internal circulation within their institutions. Permission of the Publisher is required for resale or distribution outside the institution. Permission of the Publisher is required for all other derivative works, including compilations and translations (please consult www.elsevier.com/permissions).

Electronic Storage or Usage

Permission of the Publisher is required to store or use electronically any material contained in this periodical, including any article or part of an article (please consult www.elsevier.com/permissions). Except as outlined above, no part of this publication may be reproduced, stored in a retrieval system or transmitted in any form or by any means, electronic, mechanical, photocopying, recording or otherwise, without prior written permission of the Publisher.

Notice

No responsibility is assumed by the Publisher for any injury and/or damage to persons or property as a matter of products liability, negligence or otherwise, or from any use or operation of any methods, products, instructions or ideas contained in the material herein. Because of rapid advances in the medical sciences, in particular, independent verification of diagnoses and drug dosages should be made.

Although all advertising material is expected to conform to ethical (medical) standards, inclusion in this publication does not constitute a guarantee or endorsement of the quality or value of such product or of the claims made of it by its manufacturer.

Orthopedic Clinics of North America (ISSN 0030-5898) is published quarterly by Elsevier Inc., 360 Park Avenue South, New York, NY 10010-1710. Months of issue are January, April, July, and October. Business and Editorial Offices: 1600 John F. Kennedy Blvd., Suite 1800, Philadelphia, PA 19103-2899. Customer Service Office: 3251 Riverport Lane, Maryland Heights, MO 63043. Periodicals postage paid at New York, NY and additional mailing offices. Subscription prices are $341.00 per year for (US individuals), $749.00 per year for (US institutions), $403.00 per year (Canadian individuals), $914.00 per year (Canadian institutions), $466.00 per year (international individuals), $914.00 per year (international institutions), $100.00 per year (US students), $220.00 per year (Canadian and international students). Foreign air speed delivery is included in all *Clinics* subscription prices. All prices are subject to change without notice. **POSTMASTER:** Send change of address to *Orthopedic Clinics of North America*, **Elsevier Health Sciences Division, Subscription Customer Service, 3251 Riverport Lane, Maryland Heights, MO 63043. Customer Service (orders, claims, online, change of address): Elsevier Health Sciences Division, Subscription Customer Service, 3251 Riverport Lane, Maryland Heights, MO 63043. Tel: 1-800-654-2452 (U.S. and Canada); 314-447-8871 (outside U.S. and Canada). Fax: 314-447-8029. E-mail:** journalscustomerservice-usa@elsevier.com **(for print support);** journalsonlinesupport-usa@elsevier.com **(for online support).**

Reprints. For copies of 100 or more, of articles in this publication, please contact the Commercial Reprints Department, Elsevier Inc., 360 Park Avenue South, New York, NY 10010-1710. Tel.: 212-633-3874; Fax: 212-633-3820; E-mail: reprints@elsevier.com.

Orthopedic Clinics of North America is covered in *MEDLINE/PubMed (Index Medicus), Cinahl, Excerpta Medica,* and *Cumulative Index to Nursing and Allied Health Literature.*

EDITORIAL BOARD

CONTRIBUTORS

AUTHORS

FRANK R. AVILUCEA, MD
Faculty, Level One Orthopedics, Orlando
Health, Orlando Health Orthopaedic Institute,
Orlando, Florida

BRAD D. BLANKENHORN, MD
Assistant Professor of Orthopaedics,
Department of Orthopedic Surgery, The
Warren Alpert Medical School at Brown
University, East Providence, Rhode Island

JAMES S. CHAMBERS, MD
Department of Orthopaedic Surgery and
Biomedical Engineering, Campbell Clinic,
University of Tennessee, Memphis,
Tennessee

ANNA COHEN-ROSENBLUM, MD
Assistant Professor, Department of
Orthopaedic Surgery, Louisiana State
University, New Orleans, Louisiana

QUANJUN CUI, MD
G.J. Wang Professor of Orthopaedic Surgery,
Vice Chair for Research, Department of
Orthopedic Surgery, University of Virginia,
University of Virginia School of Medicine,
Charlottesville, Virginia

KENNETH DEFONTES III, MD
Towson Orthopaedic Associates, Ruxton
Professional Center, Towson, Maryland

GRAHAM J. DEKEYSER, MD
Resident, University of Utah, Department of
Orthopaedics, Orthopaedic Center, Salt Lake
City, Utah

VAHID ENTEZARI, MD, MMSc
Orthopaedic & Rheumatologic Institute,
Department of Orthopaedic Surgery,
Cleveland Clinic, Cleveland, Ohio

JEANNE M. FRANZONE, MD
Department of Orthopaedic Surgery,
Nemours Alfred I. duPont Hospital for
Children, Wilmington, Delaware

JONATHAN A. GABOR, BS
NYU Langone Orthopedic Hospital, NYU
Langone Health, New York, New York

JUSTIN M. HALLER, MD
Associate Professor, University of Utah,
Department of Orthopaedics, Orthopaedic
Center, Salt Lake City, Utah

MICHAEL P. HORAN, MD, MS
Clinical Associate Professor of Orthopaedic
Surgery, Pediatric Orthopaedic Surgery,
Palmetto Health-USC Orthopaedic Center,
University of South Carolina, Columbia,
South Carolina

RAYMOND Y. HSU, MD
Assistant Professor of Orthopedics,
Department of Orthopedic Surgery, The
Warren Alpert Medical School at Brown
University, East Providence, Rhode
Island

DANIEL HUGHES, PhD
Medical Student MS3, Department of
Orthopaedic Surgery, University of South
Carolina School of Medicine, Columbia,
South Carolina

RICHARD IORIO, MD
Brigham and Women's Hospital, Harvard
Medical School, Boston, Massachusetts

PATRICK J. KELLAM, MD
Resident, University of Utah, Department of
Orthopaedics, Orthopaedic Center, Salt Lake
City, Utah

RICHARD W. KRUSE, DO, MBA
Department of Orthopaedic Surgery,
Nemours Alfred I. duPont Hospital for
Children, Wilmington, Delaware

MARK LAZARUS, MD
Department of Orthopaedic Surgery,
The Rothman Institute-Thomas Jefferson
University, Philadelphia, Pennsylvania

SURENA NAMDARI, MD, MSc
Associate Professor of Orthopaedic Surgery,
Director of Shoulder and Elbow Research,
Department of Orthopaedic Surgery, The
Rothman Institute, Thomas Jefferson
University, Philadelphia, Pennsylvania

SAMANTHA NINO, MD
Resident, Department of Orthopaedics,
Orlando Health, Orlando Health Orthopaedic
Institute, Orlando, Florida

JORGE A. PADILLA, MD
NYU Langone Orthopedic Hospital, NYU
Langone Health, New York, New York

JOSE M. RAMIREZ, MD, MA
Orthopedic Surgery Resident, Department of
Orthopedic Surgery, The Warren Alpert
Medical School at Brown University,
Providence, Rhode Island

HAYEEM L. RUDY, BA
NYU Langone Orthopedic Hospital, NYU
Langone Health, New York, New York

RAN SCHWARZKOPF, MD, MSc
NYU Langone Orthopedic Hospital, NYU
Langone Health, New York, New York

SUKEN A. SHAH, MD
Department of Orthopaedic Surgery,
Nemours Alfred I. duPont Hospital for
Children, Wilmington, Delaware

JEREMY T. SMITH, MD
Department of Orthopaedics, Brigham and
Women's Hospital, Harvard Medical School,
Boston, Massachusetts

SANDEEP P. SOIN, MD
Resident, Department of Orthopaedics,
Orlando Health, Orlando Health Orthopaedic
Institute, Orlando, Florida

MICHAEL A. STONE, MD
Clinical Fellow, Department of Orthopaedic
Surgery, The Rothman Institute, Thomas
Jefferson University, Philadelphia,
Pennsylvania

CARSON D. STRICKLAND, MD
Department of Orthopaedic Surgery and
Biomedical Engineering, Campbell Clinic,
University of Tennessee, Memphis,
Tennessee

JONATHAN VIGDORCHIK, MD
NYU Langone Orthopedic Hospital, NYU
Langone Health, New York, New York

MAEGEN J. WALLACE, MD
Department of Orthopaedic Surgery,
University of Nebraska Medical Center,
Children's Hospital and Medical Center,
Omaha, Nebraska

KEVIN WILLIAMS, MD
Orthopaedic Surgery Resident, PGY5,
Department of Orthopaedic Surgery,
University of South Carolina School
of Medicine, Columbia, South
Carolina

JOHN C. WU, MD
Hand Fellow, Department of Orthopaedic
Surgery and Biomedical Engineering,
Campbell Clinic, University of Tennessee,
Memphis, Tennessee

CONTENTS

Knee and Hip Reconstruction

Osteonecrosis of the femoral head most commonly arises from trauma or corticosteroid and alcohol use but is also associated with blood dyscrasias and metabolic and coagulation disorders. Initial evaluation includes a history and physical examination and plain radiographs. Early-stage osteonecrosis is best evaluated by MRI. The Ficat and Arlet classification system is the most widely used. Nonoperative treatment has been studied using bisphosphonates, anticoagulants, vasodilators, statins, and biophysical modalities. Operative treatment includes core decompression with or without adjuvants, such as autologous bone marrow, whereas total hip arthroplasty is reserved for advanced-stage osteonecrosis in older patients or those who have failed joint-preserving treatment.

Hip dislocation remains a major concern following total hip arthroplasty due to its high frequency and economic burden. This article evaluates the cost-effectiveness regarding dual mobility as an alternative to standard implant designs. A review of literature analyzing the PubMed Central database was undertaken using the following terms in the primary query: dual mobility, cost-effectiveness, cost-analysis, or economic analysis. Dual mobility systems may be a cost-effective alternative when the price of the implant does not exceed the traditional system by $1023. Dual mobility cups may be an essential component for the future success of value-based total hip arthroplasty.

Trauma

The incidence of osteoporotic fracture is increasing with the aging US population. Because osteoporosis leads to a decrease in bone mineral density with a decrease in both trabecular and cortical bones, osteoporotic fracture presents fixation challenges with standard plate and screw constructs. Locked plating has been developed to create a fixed-angle plate-screw construct that is more resistant to failure in osteoporotic bone. Endosteal replacement, additional plates, and cement augmentation have all been demonstrated to further supplement osteoporotic fracture fixation. Technologies on the horizon to treat osteoporotic fracture include SMV screws, hydroxyapatite-coated implants, and far cortical locking screws.

reduction and hardware fixation. Loss of fixation and varus collapse continue to be problems despite the utilization of modern locking plate fixation. A clearer understanding of predictors of fixation failure and the encouraging early results of reverse total shoulder arthroplasty (RTSA) have resulted in increased utilization of RTSA for the primary treatment of proximal humerus fractures.

Osteopenia and osteoporosis are common in older adults and are associated with increased risk of fragility fractures. Vitamin D deficiency caused by chronic disease, poor nutrition, and inadequate sun exposure affects bone quality. Chronic rotator cuff tears can deteriorate the bone mineral density of the greater tuberosity and have been linked to reduced anchor pullout strength and high re-tear rate after repair especially in older patients with larger tear size. This article summarizes the current evidence on rotator cuff tear and bone quality and provides treatment strategies for rotator cuff repair in patients with poor bone quality.

Foot and Ankle

As the geriatric population and associated ankle fractures continues to increase, fracture surgeons should be prepared to surgically manage osteoporotic ankle fractures. There are abundant challenges in management, soft tissue care, and fixation of ankle fractures with poor bone quality especially in elderly patients who have difficulty limiting weight bearing. This article summarizes several different surgical techniques that can be used to optimize outcomes of these fractures.

Vitamin D deficiency affects nearly one-sixth of the world's population and is common in patients undergoing foot and ankle surgery. Vitamin D is critical for calcium homeostasis and plays an important role in the maintenance of bone health. Patients undergoing foot and ankle procedures can be evaluated preoperatively with vitamin D level testing, and deficiencies can be addressed with either preoperative or postoperative supplementation. Current data suggest that patients with adequate vitamin D levels may have better outcomes, but the details are not yet clear. Vitamin D supplementation is well tolerated with rare side effects.

SURGICAL CONSIDERATIONS FOR OSTEOPOROSIS, OSTEOPENIA, AND VITAMIN D DEFICIENCY

SERIES OF RELATED INTEREST

Clinics in Podiatric Medicine and Surgery
Clinics in Sports Medicine
Foot and Ankle Clinics
Hand Clinics
Physical Medicine and Rehabilitation Clinics of North America

PREFACE

Surgical Considerations for Osteoporosis, Osteopenia, and Vitamin D Deficiency

Osteoporosis, osteopenia, and the importance of adequate vitamin D have been recognized for many years, but their effects on orthopedic injuries and conditions have not been completely defined, and testing for and treating vitamin D deficiency are not currently performed routinely for most orthopedic patients, even though vitamin D supplementation is inexpensive and simple and has an excellent safety profile.

Authors in this issue of *Orthopedic Clinics of North America* discuss treatment considerations for fractures in osteoporotic bones. Drs Cohen-Rosenblum and Cui discuss operative treatment of femoral head osteonecrosis, including core decompression, with or without adjuvants such as autologous bone marrow, and total hip arthroplasty. Dr Rudy and colleagues describe the use of dual-mobility cups in hip arthroplasty to prevent dislocation and suggest that use of this component may be a cost-effective measure.

Drs DeKeyser, Kellam, and Haller provide a thorough overview of fixation techniques for osteoporotic fractures, including locked plating and cement augmentation, while Drs Nino, Soin, and Avilucea point out the need for consideration of vitamin D deficiency in patients with fracture nonunions of uncertain cause. As noted by Dr Wu, distal radial fractures are frequent in older individuals and often are the first clinical sign of osteoporosis, allowing pharmacotherapy when appropriate to reduce the risk of future fragility fractures. Drs Stone and Namdari emphasize the challenges of treatment of proximal humeral fractures in osteoporotic patients and suggest that reverse total shoulder arthroplasty may be a good alternative to standard fixation techniques. While the topics of bone quality and fragility fractures have been well studied, their relationship with rotator cuff tear and repair has received less attention. Drs Entezari and Lazarus summarize the current evidence on the effect of rotator cuff tears on bone quality and provide treatment strategies for rotator cuff repair in patients with poor bone quality. The frequency of foot and ankle trauma continues to increase with the increase of elderly patients in the United States. Drs Hsu, Ramirez, and Blankenhorn provide several surgical techniques that can be used to optimize outcomes of these fractures, while Drs DeFontes and Smith note that patients with adequate vitamin D levels appear to have better outcomes, and preoperative vitamin D testing can allow deficiencies to be treated.

The importance of vitamin D in the growth and development of children's bones has been recognized for over a century, and the association of vitamin D deficiency and rickets was delineated in the *Journal of Pediatrics* in 1968; 50 years later, the frequency of nutritional rickets is on the rise. Drs Horan, Williams, and Hughes review the main areas in which vitamin D affects pediatric patients and highlight some of the areas where future research is being directed. Although not associated with vitamin D deficiency, osteogenesis imperfecta (OI) results in some similar conditions (eg, brittle bones, fractures, deformities of the spine and extremities). Dr Franzone and colleagues describe the presentation and management considerations for patients with OI.

As these authors have noted, patients with osteoporosis, osteopenia, or vitamin D deficiency pose a challenge for orthopedists. Pharmacotherapy (eg, vitamin D supplementation, bisphosphonates) can help reduce the risk of fracture and deformity, and a variety of techniques are available for treatment when such injuries or deformities occur.

Frederick M. Azar, MD
Campbell Clinic
University of Tennessee–Campbell Clinic
Department of Orthopaedic Surgery
1211 Union Avenue, Suite 510
Memphis, TN 38104, USA

E-mail address:
fazar@campbellclinic.com

Orthop Clin N Am 50 (2019) xi
https://doi.org/10.1016/j.ocl.2019.01.001
0030-5898/19/© 2019 Published by Elsevier Inc.

Knee and Hip Reconstruction

Osteonecrosis of the Femoral Head

Anna Cohen-Rosenblum, MD[a], Quanjun Cui, MD[b],*

KEYWORDS

- Femoral head osteonecrosis • Corticosteroid • Core decompression • Stem cell
- Total hip arthroplasty

KEY POINTS

- Osteonecrosis of the femoral head most commonly arises from trauma or corticosteroid and alcohol use but is also associated with blood dyscrasias and metabolic and coagulation disorders.
- Although initial evaluation should include a thorough history and physical examination and plain radiographs of the hip and pelvis, early-stage osteonecrosis is best evaluated by MRI.
- Operative treatment includes core decompression with or without adjuvants, such as autologous bone marrow, whereas total hip arthroplasty is reserved for advanced-stage osteonecrosis in older patients or those who have failed joint-preserving treatment.

INTRODUCTION

Osteonecrosis of the femoral head (ONFH) is a devastating condition affecting patients in the third to fifth decades of life that usually progresses to femoral head collapse, often leading to total hip arthroplasty (THA).[1–4] Although the etiology, pathogenesis, diagnosis, and treatment of ONFH have been studied extensively, there is no clear consensus as to its exact origin. ONFH is "not a specific disease, but rather the end result of various conditions, ultimately, with impairment of blood to the femoral head."[5] This article provides an updated overview of the potential etiology and risk factors for ONFH as well as diagnosis, classification systems, and nonoperative and operative treatments.

ETIOLOGY AND RISK FACTORS

ONFH is essentially bone cell death from compromised microvascular circulation believed the result of

1. Mechanical vascular interruption
2. Intravascular occlusion
3. Extravascular compression[6,7]

These processes can be the result of trauma, corticosteroids, alcohol use, blood dyscrasias, and miscellaneous factors.

Trauma

Trauma leads to ONFH by mechanically disrupting the vascular supply to the femoral head.[2] This occurs when the main blood supply to the adult femoral head (medial circumflex femoral

---

Disclosure: Dr A. Cohen-Rosenblum has no conflicts of interest to declare. Dr Q. Cui or an immediate family member serves as a paid consultant to Exactech; has received research or institutional support from National Institute of Health, Department of Defense, United States, and Exactech; serves as a board member, owner, officer, or committee member of Association Research Circulation Osseous, Virginia Orthopaedic Society, *Journal of Arthroplasty*, *World Journal of Orthopedics*, and *Journal of Orthopaedic Research*; and has received royalties from Elsevier.

[a] Department of Orthopaedic Surgery, Louisiana State University, 1542 Tulane Avenue, New Orleans, LA 70112, USA; [b] Department of Orthopedic Surgery, University of Virginia, University of Virginia School of Medicine, 400 Ray C. Hunt Drive, #300, Charlottesville, VA 22903, USA
* Corresponding author.
E-mail address: QC4Q@hscmail.mcc.virginia.edu

artery) is disrupted due to a femoral head fracture, displaced femoral neck fracture, or hip dislocation.[8] Fractures occurring further away from the medial circumflex femoral artery in the intertrochanteric or subtrochanteric regions rarely lead to ONFH, although it is possible for this to develop as a result of antegrade intramedullary femoral nailing in a skeletally mature individual.[8–10] Nondisplaced femoral neck fractures treated with closed reduction and percutaneous pinning can also lead to ONFH, with a recent database study showing a 10% conversion rate to arthroplasty at 5 years.[11] In the pediatric population, ONFH can be caused by antegrade intramedullary nailing from a piriform entry point.[12]

Corticosteroids

Corticosteroids are considered the most common cause of atraumatic ONFH, and the exact mechanism is unknown.[13] A 2015 meta-analysis by Mont and colleagues[14] found a statistically significant association between high-dose corticosteroid use (>20 mg prednisone-equivalents per day) and ONFH, but cases have been reported from long-term and short-term doses and after oral, intravenous, topical, and intraarticular application.[13–18] The most commonly accepted theory surrounding corticosteroids and ONFH involves fat accumulation in marrow, leading to increased intraosseous hypertension and decreased blood flow.[1,6,19,20]

This concept has been extrapolated into a multiple-hit theory by which corticosteroids alter bone homeostasis, injure bone cells, impair blood flow, and suppress bone cell precursors in susceptible patients.[1,13,20] In support of the multiple-hit theory, Wang and colleagues[19] found increased differentiation of pluripotential stem cells into adipocytes and reduced expression of type I collagen and osteocalcin messenger RNA in an animal model. Corticosteroids inhibit angiogenesis and promote a hypercoagulable state, which could contribute to the formation of intravascular thrombosis leading to ONFH.[13] Also, studies have investigated whether there is a genetic susceptibility to corticosteroid-induced ONFH.[1,20,21] Because not all patients receiving corticosteroids develop ONFH, it is most likely due to a combination of factors, including genetic susceptibility, dosage, and underlying condition.[1,13,14,20]

Alcohol

The connection between alcohol use and ONFH has been known for almost a century, and, as with corticosteroids, the exact mechanism is unknown.[22] Animal studies of bone marrow treated with alcohol have shown increased pressure and adipogenesis and decreased hematopoiesis, which could lead to osteocyte injury and ONFH.[22–24] There seems to be a dose-response relationship; however, there is no established threshold beyond which patients are proved more at risk.[22] Given the relatively low prevalence of ONFH among all alcohol users, there is likely a multifactorial relationship between ONFH, genetic susceptibility, environmental factors, and medical comorbidities.[6,22,25]

Blood Dyscrasias

Blood dyscrasias cause ONFH by intravascular occlusion.[1,2,6,20,26,27] ONFH frequently occurs in sickle cell disease, in which the pathologic sickled erythrocytes obstruct the vessels to the femoral head.[6,26] Data from Hernigou and colleagues[28] suggest a more rapid clinical progression of ONFH from sickle cell disease compared with other nontraumatic causes. Patients with polycythemia vera, a myeloproliferative neoplasm causing erythrocytosis, are at risk for ONFH due to thrombosis.[2,29] Hemophilia (a bleeding disorder caused by a lack of clotting factors) has been reported to cause ONFH via intravascular occlusion from recurrent intraosseous hemorrhage.[27] Finally, genetic defects leading to hypercoagulable states (factor V Leiden mutation, protein C/S deficiency, increased von Willebrand factor, and increased lipoprotein levels) are hypothesized to cause ONFH from intravascular thrombosis.[2,6,20,30]

Miscellaneous

Many other risk factors have been associated with ONFH. Gaucher disease is a metabolic disorder in which an enzyme deficiency causes abnormal accumulation of glucocerebroside in macrophages, which infiltrate the bone marrow causing compression and vascular compromise.[31] A study of patients with Gaucher disease and ONFH found that it was more prevalent in patients who had a prior splenectomy.[32] Caisson disease, also referred to as decompression syndrome or the bends, occurs when gaseous bubbles enter tissues after exposure to rapid changes in barometric pressure, including mine or tunnel work, deep sea diving, or riding in an unpressurized aircraft.[33,34] Dysbaric osteonecrosis occurs when gas bubbles enter the medullary canal and constrict blood flow.[33]

HIV also has been associated with ONFH, but it is unclear whether it is from a disease-specific mechanism, antiretrovirals, or other confounding risk factors.[1,35] Similarly, systemic lupus erythematosus has been associated with ONFH through the disease process itself, corticosteroid use, cytotoxic medications, and vasculitis.[36–38] Radiation treatment is also believed a risk factor for ONFH, but there has been no determination of a dose-response relationship or explanation for why unilateral ONFH can occur after equal radiation exposure to both femoral heads.[2,20,39] ONFH has also been linked to pregnancy, inflammatory bowel disease, malignant tumors, gout, and smoking.[2,20]

DIAGNOSIS AND CLASSIFICATION SYSTEMS

Physical Examination

After obtaining a thorough patient history, a physical examination is helpful in confirming a suspected diagnosis of ONFH. Patients may complain of pain in the groin, buttock, or knee. Examination signs of ONFH include pain with internal rotation of the hip. Severely restricted hip internal rotation may indicate femoral head collapse.[3]

Imaging

If history and physical examination findings are suspicious for ONFH, plain radiography is the next step in diagnosis. Although very early

ONFH may be undetectable on plain radiography,[2,40] early ONFH shows, on anteroposterior (AP) pelvis and frog lateral views, cystic and/or sclerotic changes in the femoral head (**Fig. 1**). The term, *crescent sign*, describes an area of subchondral lucency in the femoral head that indicates subchondral fracture due to bone necrosis and subsequent attempts at repair (**Fig. 2**).[2,3,40] ONFH at a later stage shows femoral head flattening, collapse, and degenerative changes (**Fig. 3**).

MRI is the modality of choice for patients with a suspicious history and physical examination with normal radiographs. It is 99% sensitive and specific for detecting early ONFH, which usually presents as an area of low-intensity signal on T1-weighted and high-intensity signal on T2-weighted images (see **Fig. 1C, D**).[2,3,40] Bone marrow edema and a joint effusion also may be present.[40]

The later stages of ONFH are better followed using plain radiography and, in some cases, CT.[40] CT is useful for evaluating patients with a suspected subchondral fracture, which may not be seen on MRI.[40] Technetium bone scans and PET scans have also been used to evaluate ONFH but are not as sensitive as MRI.[2,40–42] In conclusion, plain radiography should be used

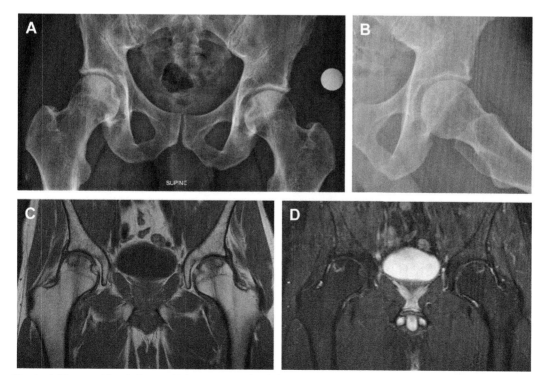

Fig. 1. A 50 year-old male heavy drinker presented with bilateral groin pain and radiographic findings of femoral head sclerosis on AP (*A*) and frog lateral (*B*) views. MRI showed (*C*) T1 hypointense and (*D*) T2 hyperintense signal of the necrotic lesions of the femoral heads bilaterally.

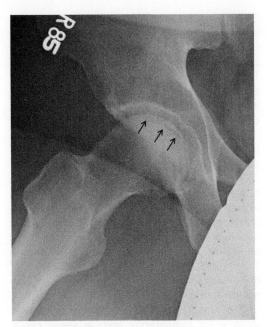

Fig. 2. The crescent sign describes an area of subchondral lucency in the femoral head (*arrows*) that indicates subchondral fracture.

for initial evaluation of suspected ONFH as well as after disease progression in the later stages, with MRI to be used in the setting of normal radiographs with suspicious history and/or examination findings.

Classification Systems

Multiple classification systems have been developed for ONFH. This section focuses on the 4 most commonly used systems: Ficat and Arlet, University of Pennsylvania/Steinberg, Association Research Circulation Osseous (ARCO), and the Japanese Orthopaedic Association.[43,44] In addition, the method devised by

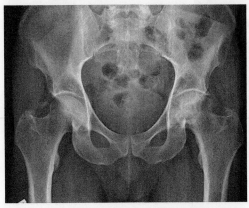

Fig. 3. AP pelvis view shows a collapsed left femoral head with arthritic changes of the hip joint.

Kerboul to measure osteonecrotic lesions is discussed.[45]

The Ficat and Arlet classification system was first developed in the 1960s and is based on clinical symptoms, radiographic findings, and uptake on bone scan.[41] It is the most commonly used classification system as well as the most straightforward but does not account for size or location of the osteonecrotic lesion, which are now considered important factors predicting treatment outcomes.[43] Stage 0 is preclinical, with no findings on imaging expect for reduced uptake on bone scan. Stage I is preradiographic, with clinical symptoms and increased uptake on bone scan. Stage II involves sclerotic or cystic changes on radiographs without femoral head flattening or crescent sign. Stage III involves the radiographic crescent sign with preserved joint space, whereas stage IV is defined as femoral head flattening and arthritic changes of the hip joint.[41,43]

The University of Pennsylvania/Steinberg classification system was developed in the 1980s and incorporates MRI findings as well as size and articular involvement of the osteonecrotic lesion.[44] As with the Ficat and Arlet system, stage 0 is normal or nondiagnostic imaging. Stage I is normal radiographs with abnormal MRI and/or bone scan, with a subclassification of A, B, or C based on the percentage of femoral head affected by the lesion. Stage II involves cystic or sclerotic changes in the femoral head, also subclassified by percentage of femoral head involved. Stage III involves a crescent sign without flattening of the femoral head, subclassified by percentage of articular surface involvement. Stage IV involves flattening of the femoral head that is subclassified by percentage of femoral head surface involvement and millimeters of depression. Stage V involves joint-space narrowing or acetabular changes, subclassified into mild, moderate, and severe. Stage VI is defined as advanced degenerative radiographic changes.[44]

The ARCO classification system was developed in the early 1990s based on the University of Pennsylvania system but with additional 4 subclassifications to reflect location of the lesion, percentage of femoral head involvement, length of crescent, and percentage of collapse.[43,44] There are 5 total stages:

- 0 (normal imaging findings)
- I (positive findings on bone scan or MRI)
- II (abnormal radiographic findings with sclerotic and/or cystic changes with abnormal MRI, CT, and/or bone scan findings)

- III (crescent sign and/or femoral head flattening)
- IV (degenerative radiographic changes)[44]

This system was found unnecessarily complicated and is not used as frequently as the Ficat and Arlet or University of Pennsylvania systems.[43,44]

The Japanese Orthopaedic Association classification system was developed in the late 1980s. It is based on the Ficat and Arlet system but subdivides stages II and III according to the lesion's type and location seen on AP radiographs.[4,43,44] It does not include Ficat and Arlet stages 0, I, and IV. Due to concerns regarding its ambiguity and lack of classification of the early and late stages of ONFH, it is used mostly in Japan.[43]

Kerboul and colleagues[43,45] developed a method of measuring the size of osteonecrotic lesions to predict treatment outcome. They measured the angles encompassing the lesions on AP and lateral radiographs and hypothesized that patients with a sum less than 180° had improved outcomes compared with those with a sum greater than 230°.[43] Ha and colleagues[45] adapted this method for use with MRI and found that patients with a combined necrotic angle less than 190° had a low risk of collapse compared with those with a combined necrotic angle greater than 240°, over at least 5 years of follow-up.

Although it is interesting to compare these different methods of classifying ONFH, ultimately the most useful system for the clinician is both easy to use and reliable at predicting clinical outcome. Therefore, it is not surprising that the Ficat and Arlet system remains the most commonly cited in the orthopedic literature.[43]

TREATMENT
Nonoperative
There are many nonoperative treatments available for ONFH, most with limited supporting data. Activity modification with restricted weight bearing is often used for symptomatic relief, but does not seem to have any effect on disease progression.[46,47] Pharmacologic and biophysical treatment of ONFH is mainly experimental at this time and consists of bisphosphonates, anticoagulants, vasodilators, statins, and biophysical modalities.

Bisphosphonates, which reduce osteoclast activity, theoretically may prevent femoral head collapse in patients with early ONFH by inhibiting the increased bone turnover that occurs around the necrotic region.[1,4] The results of human studies are inconclusive.[48,49] A 2016 meta-

analysis of 5 randomized clinical trials found no statistically significant improvement in ONFH patients treated with bisphosphonates,[50] and a 2018 meta-analysis that included both animal and human studies found that although there was improvement in animal model outcomes, similar results were not found for humans.[51] Given that bisphosphonates can have adverse effects, such as atypical proximal femur fractures and osteonecrosis of the jaw, more definitive research is needed before routinely recommending this treatment of early-stage ONFH.[50]

Because one of the proposed mechanisms for the pathophysiology of ONFH is intravascular occlusion, anticoagulants and vasodilators theoretically could delay or even reverse disease progression, but supporting data are limited.[4] A prospective study of 30 hips with ONFH associated with coagulopathy treated with the anticoagulant enoxaparin showed 53% had not progressed beyond Ficat and Arlet stages I and II, which was improved compared with historical controls.[52] Animal models with steroid-induced ONFH have shown improved femoral head perfusion after treatment with enoxaparin and ginkgo biloba extract (a vasodilator) as well as sildenafil.[53,54] It remains to be seen whether these results can be replicated in human studies and whether these medications would be indicated only for coagulopathy-related ONFH.

One potential etiology for corticosteroid-induced ONFH is fat accumulation in marrow, leading to increased intraosseous hypertension and decreased blood flow. Statins, which lower lipid levels by blocking cholesterol synthesis, could potentially prevent these effects.[55] A chicken model with steroid-induced ONFH treated with lovastatin was found to decrease adipogenesis and bone death, and marrow cells treated with lovastatin were shown to have increased osteoblastic gene expression.[56] Retrospective studies of lower-level evidence have shown equivocal results. One study examined more than 3000 renal transplants and found no statistically significant relationship between statin use and decreased risk of ONFH, and another, smaller study examined patients taking both statins and high-dose steroids and found a 1% incidence of ONFH after a mean 7.5 years' follow-up with no control group.[57,58] More studies of a higher level of evidence must be performed to provide more conclusive data and remove confounding factors.

In addition to these pharmacologic treatments, various biophysical treatments have been applied to ONFH, including extracorporeal shock wave therapy, electrical stimulation, and hyperbaric oxygen.[4] Wang and colleagues[59] performed a randomized clinical trial of ARCO stages I to III ONFH patients undergoing shock wave treatments compared with core decompression and nonvascularized fibular grafting and found improved pain and Harris hip scores and slower disease progression. A recent systematic review of electrical stimulation therapy for ONFH found modestly encouraging results of 10 studies, none of which was level I evidence.[60] Hyperbaric oxygen therapy, which theoretically reduces cellular ischemia by increasing the extracellular oxygen concentration, was also found to have encouraging results for early-stage ONFH patients in a 2017 systematic review.[4,61] At this time, the use of nonoperative pharmacologic and biophysical treatment modalities for ONFH is limited to the experimental realm and/or early stages of the disease.

Operative

For later-stage ONFH or patients who have had unsuccessful nonoperative treatment, the next step is consideration of operative management. The most common operative interventions are discussed, including core decompression, bone grafting, and THA, with a brief mention of procedures that were more common historically.

Core decompression

Core decompression is a joint-preserving operative technique that aims to improve blood flow to the femoral head by decreasing intraosseous pressure, thereby potentially delaying or preventing THA.[4,62] Traditional core decompression is performed using a trephine to remove an 8-mm to 10-mm core from the osteonecrotic lesion in the femoral head, while avoiding penetrating the articular surface (Fig. 4A).[1,62] This method has been found to have satisfactory results in precollapse ONFH with smaller lesions (involving <15% of the femoral head), with the potential disadvantages of intraoperative cartilage penetration and postoperative subtrochanteric femur fracture.[62] These complications may be avoided by using the multiple drilling technique, in which small guide wires are passed percutaneously multiple times through the lesion (see Fig. 4B). This technique is also recommended for larger lesions that are at risk for collapse.[4,62] Both methods are followed by postoperative weight-bearing restrictions for 6 weeks.[62]

Core decompression may also be combined with adjuvant substances, including autologous bone marrow aspirate containing mesenchymal stem cells (MSCs), various growth factors, and tantalum rods.[3,62–65] MSCs are hypothesized to improve osteogenesis by differentiating into osteoblasts as well as secreting growth factors that may stimulate repair of the osteonecrotic lesion and prevent femoral head collapse.[7,65] Hernigou and Beaujean[63] prospectively followed 189 hips treated with core decompression and autologous bone marrow aspirate concentrate obtained from the anterior iliac crest (Fig. 5) and found that 6% (9/145) of patients treated precollapse and 57% (25/44) of those treated postcollapse required THA at a mean of 7 years

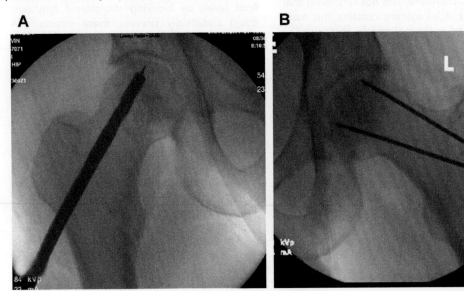

Fig. 4. Core decompression can be performed (A) using a trephine to remove an 8-mm to 10-mm core from the osteonecrotic lesion in the femoral head or (B) using small guide wires to pass multiple times through the lesion.

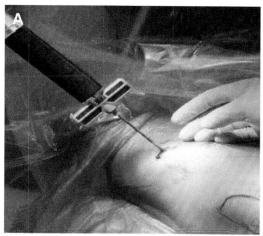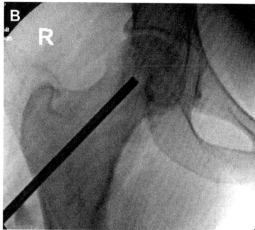

Fig. 5. (A) Autologous bone marrow aspirated from the anterior iliac crest is concentrated and then (B) delivered to the necrotic lesion site through the core decompression tract.

follow-up. By analyzing the bone marrow samples, they also found that patients with a greater number of transplanted progenitor cells had improved outcomes.[63]

Adjuvant growth factors, such as bone morphogenetic proteins and angiogenic growth factors, also have the potential to encourage bone regeneration in osteonecrotic lesions, but the question remains as to the ideal method of delivery.[66] Bone morphogenetic protein delivery on various types of scaffolding has been described in multiple animal models, and a prospective study by Houdek and colleagues[66,67] of precollapse steroid-induced ONFH patients treated with core decompression augmented with MSCs from autologous bone marrow aspirate and additional growth factors from platelet-rich plasma found that more than 90% of patients were without collapse at a minimum of 2 years' follow-up. A 2017 meta-analysis of 11 randomized controlled trials with 507 participants found improved results with core decompression combined with autologous bone marrow stem cells, but to truly understand the effect of these substances, more research should be done comparing core decompression done with and without specific adjuvants.[68]

Tantalum implants were theorized to potentially prevent femoral head collapse and encourage healing through structural support and osteoinductive properties, but short-term results and histologic analysis of retrieved implants during conversion to THA have not been encouraging.[3]

Bone grafting

Bone grafting has been used to treat ONFH since the mid-twentieth century and is theorized

to prevent femoral head collapse by providing structural support.[69] Nonvascularized cortical autograft or allograft has been inserted into the osteonecrotic femoral head lesions using the Phemister technique (using the core decompression tract accessed through the lateral proximal femur), the lightbulb technique (via a cortical window in the femoral neck accessed through an anterior arthrotomy), and the trapdoor technique (via a flap of articular cartilage accessed through surgical dislocation).[4,70] These procedures are generally indicated for small to medium-sized lesions in younger patients seeking to delay or prevent THA, with lower-level supporting evidence.[1]

Vascularized bone grafting is thought to combine the structural support of nonvascularized bone graft with increased healing potential from a revived blood supply.[69] Vascularized bone graft can be harvested from a patient's fibula, iliac crest, and greater trochanter.[69,71,72] Vascularized fibular graft is the most studied of these procedures and is performed by exposing the proximal femur using an anterolateral approach, mobilizing a branch of the lateral femoral circumflex artery, reaming the necrotic area of the femoral head, harvesting a section of fibula, and anastomosing the fibular vessels to the donor vessels mobilized around the femur.[71] This complex procedure has multiple potential complications, including donor site morbidity, venous thromboembolism, and infection.[71] According to its proponents, it is indicated for younger symptomatic patients with ONFH (including postcollapse) or precollapse patients between 20 years and 50 years old.[71,72] A 2017 randomized clinical trial by Cao and colleagues[73] found that vascularized free fibular graft had improved vascularity and decreased progression of ONFH compared with core decompression, but no difference was found in conversion to THA at 3 years of follow-up.

Total hip arthroplasty

For patients with advanced ONFH or failure of joint-preserving operative treatments, THA is an attractive option with excellent outcomes in terms of pain relief and survivorship.[1,4,74] Although earlier studies of THA in the setting of ONFH had poorer outcomes with high rates of loosening, studies performed after the adoption of highly cross-linked polyethylene, uncemented femoral stems, and fourth-generation ceramic bearings have found outcomes that are essentially equivalent to that of primary THA performed for degenerative osteoarthritis.[1,74,75] Studies have shown increased rates of intraoperative complications and operative times in THA performed in ONFH patients who have undergone prior treatment with femoral osteotomies and vascularized bone grafting, but these patients can still benefit greatly in terms of pain relief and function.[74,75] Care must be taken when performing THA in ONFH patients because the bone may be of poor quality due to the patient's underlying condition, corticosteroid use, and/or decreased preoperative weight-bearing.[3]

Less Common Procedures

ONFH has also been treated with hemiresurfacing, total resurfacing, proximal femur rotational osteotomy, resection arthroplasty, and arthrodesis.[1,4,76–78] Hemiresurfacing, in which the femoral head is resurfaced and the acetabulum is left alone, was proposed as a way to delay THA in younger patients but has a fairly high rate of conversion to THA due to acetabular wear.[1,76] Total hip resurfacing was more popular in the early 2000s but has fallen out of favor due to concerns regarding the metal-on-metal bearing surface as well as risk of femoral neck fracture.[1,3] Proximal femur rotational osteotomy for ONFH is performed to rotate the necrotic lesion away from the weight-bearing area.[4] This procedure is performed mostly in Asia in younger, low–body mass index patients with early ONFH and can lead to complications involving nonunion and hardware failure as well as increased difficulty during conversion to THA.[1] Resection arthroplasty and arthrodesis are rarely performed today for ONFH given the excellent outcomes from THA, but resection arthroplasty may be indicated in the setting of infection and severe medical comorbidities.[77,78]

When determining the appropriate treatment of ONFH, consideration should be given to patient age, disease stage (including lesion size and location), and/or Kerboul angle.[79] For earlier-stage, precollapse small lesions in younger patients or asymptomatic patients of any age, consider nonoperative therapy as first-line treatment. Older postcollapse patients should be given the option of THA. If nonoperative therapy fails in younger early-stage patients with a lower Kerboul angle, consider joint-preserving operative techniques, such as core decompression with or without adjuvants and vascularized or nonvascularized bone grafting. Failure of nonoperative therapy in older precollapse patients or those with a larger Kerboul angle should also be given the option of THA. Any patient who has failed operative treatment with joint-preserving procedures also should be considered for THA.

SUMMARY

ONFH is a complex condition that is not fully understood. It most commonly arises from trauma or corticosteroid and alcohol use but is also associated with a variety of other risk factors, including blood dyscrasias and metabolic and coagulation disorders. Initial evaluation of ONFH should include a thorough history and physical examination as well as plain radiographs of the hip and pelvis. Early-stage ONFH is best evaluated by MRI, and CT scan can be helpful in identifying subchondral fractures. Many classification systems have been developed to categorize the different stages of ONFH, but the simplest and most widely used is the Ficat and Arlet system, and, for treatment purposes, patients can be divided into prefemoral and postfemoral head collapse. Nonoperative treatment of ONFH has been studied using bisphosphonates, anticoagulants, vasodilators, statins, and biophysical modalities, but more research should be done to determine their efficacy and safety. Operative treatment consists of joint-preserving procedures, such as core decompression with or without adjuvants, with THA reserved for advanced-stage ONFH in older patients or those who have failed joint-preserving treatment. Research involving stem cells and growth factors shows promise in clarifying both the etiology and treatment of this devastating disease.

REFERENCES

1. Mont M, Cherian J, Sierra R, et al. Nontraumatic osteonecrosis of the femoral head: where do we stand today? A ten-year update. J Bone Joint Surg Am 2015;97:1604–27.

2. Choi H, Steinberg M, Cheng E. Osteonecrosis of the femoral head: diagnosis and classification systems. Curr Rev Musculoskelet Med 2015;8:210–20.

3. Zalavras C, Lieberman J. Osteonecrosis of the femoral head: evaluation and treatment. J Am Acad Orthop Surg 2014;22:455–64.

4. Banerjee S, Issa K, Pivec R, et al. Osteonecrosis of the hip: treatment options and outcomes. Orthop Clin North Am 2013;44:463–76.

5. Plancher K, Razi A. Management of osteonecrosis of the femoral head. Orthop Clin N Am 1997; 28(3):461–77.

6. Shah K, Racine J, Jones L, et al. Pathophysiology and risk factors for osteonecrosis. Curr Rev Musculoskelet Med 2015;8:201–9.

7. Cui Q, Botchwey E. Treatment of precollapse osteonecrosis using stem cells and growth factors. Clin Orthop Relat Res 2011;469:2665–9.

8. Steppacher SD, Haefeli PC, Anwander H, et al. Traumatic avascular necrosis of the femoral head. In: Koo K, Mont M, Jones L, editors. Osteonecrosis. Berlin: Springer; 2014. p. 101–12.

9. Graves R, Sands K. Avascular necrosis of the femoral head following intramedullary nailing of the femur in a skeletally mature young adult: a case report. Am J Orthop 2008;37(6):319–22.

10. Wu C, Yu C, Hsieh C, et al. Femoral head avascular necrosis after interlocking nail of a femoral shaft fracture in a male adult: a case report. Arch Orthop Trauma Surg 2008;128:399–402.

11. Kahlenberg C, Richardson S, Schairer W, et al. Rates and risk factors of conversion hip arthroplasty after closed reduction percutaneous hip pinning for femoral neck fractures—a population analysis. J Arthroplasty 2018;33:771–6.

12. MacNeil JA, Francis A, El-Hawary R. A systematic review of rigid, locked, intramedullary nail insertion sites and avascular necrosis of the femoral head in the skeletally immature. J Pediatr Orthop 2011;31: 377–80.

13. Lee EY, Lee YJ. Glucocorticoids (as an etiologic factor). In: Koo K, Mont M, Jones L, editors. Osteonecrosis. Berlin: Springer; 2014. p. 81–90.

14. Mont M, Pivec R, Banerjee S, et al. High-dose corticosteroid use and risk of hip osteonecrosis: meta-analysis and systematic literature review. J Arthroplasty 2015;30:1506–12.

15. McKee M, Waddell J, Kudo P. Osteonecrosis of the femoral head in men following short-course corticosteroid therapy: a report of 15 case. Can Med Assoc J 2001;164(2):205–6.

16. Takahashi H, Tsuji H, Honma M, et al. Femoral head osteonecrosis after long-term corticosteroid treatment in a psoriasis patient. J Dermatol 2012; 39(10):887–8.

17. Felten R, Messer L, Moreau P, et al. Osteonecrosis of the femoral head linked to topical steroids for skin bleaching: a case report. Ann Intern Med 2014;161(10):763–4.

18. Yamamoto T, Schneider R, Iwamoto Y, et al. Rapid destruction of the femoral head after a single intra-articular injection of corticosteroid into the hip joint. J Rheumatol 2006;33:1701–4.

19. Wang G, Cui Q, Balian G. The pathogenesis and prevention of steroid induced osteonecrosis. Clin Orthop Relat Res 2000;370:295–310.

20. Seamon J, Keller T, Saleh J, et al. The pathogenesis of nontraumatic osteonecrosis. Arthritis 2012;2012: 601763.

21. Kaneshiro Y, Oda Y, Iwakiri K, et al. Low hepatic cytochrome P450 3A activity is a risk for corticosteroid-induced osteonecrosis. Clin Pharmacol Ther 2006;80(4):396–402.

22. Fukushima W, Hirota Y. Alcohol. In: Koo K, Mont M, Jones L, editors. Osteonecrosis. Berlin: Springer; 2014. p. 95–9.

23. Wang Y, Li Y, Mao K, et al. Alcohol-induced adipogenesis in bone and marrow: a possible mechanism for osteonecrosis. Clin Orthop Relat Res 2003;410: 213–24.

24. Wang Y, Yin L, Li Y, et al. Preventive effects of puerarin on alcohol-induced osteonecrosis. Clin Orthop Relat Res 2008;466:1059–67.

25. Gold E, Cangemi P. Incidence and pathogenesis of alcohol-induced osteonecrosis of the femoral head. Clin Orthop Relat Res 1979;143:222–6.

26. Hernigou P, Daltro G. Osteonecrosis in sickle-cell disease. In: Koo K, Mont M, Jones L, editors. Osteonecrosis. Berlin: Springer; 2014. p. 125–31.

27. Kilcoyne R, Nuss R. Femoral head osteonecrosis in a child with hemophilia. Arthritis Rheum 1999;42(7): 1550–1.

28. Hernigou P, Habibi A, Bachir D, et al. The natural history of asymptomatic osteonecrosis of the femoral head in adults with sickle cell disease. J Bone Joint Surg 2006;88-A(12):2565–72.

29. Tefferi A, Barbui T. Polycythemia vera and essential thrombocythemia: 2015 update on diagnosis, risk-stratification, and management. Am J Hematol 2015;90:163–73.

30. Zalavras C, Dailiana Z, Elisaf M, et al. Potential aetiological factors concerning the development of osteonecrosis of the femoral head. Eur J Clin Invest 2000;30(3):215–21.

31. Yoo JJ. Autoimmune disease and other risk factors. In: Koo K, Mont M, Jones L, editors. Osteonecrosis. Berlin: Springer; 2014. p. 133–9.

32. Rodrigue S, Rosenthal D, Barton N, et al. Risk factors for osteonecrosis in patients with Type I Gaucher's disease. Clin Orthop Relat Res 1999; 362:201–7.

33. Sharareh B, Schwarzkopf R. Dysbaric osteonecrosis: a literature review of pathophysiology, clinical presentation, and management. Clin J Sport Med 2015;25:153–61.

34. Lehner C, Adams W, Dubielzig R, et al. Dysbaric osteonecrosis in divers and caisson workers. Clin Orthop Relat Res 1997;344:320–32.

35. Borges A, Hoy J, Florence E, et al. Antiretrovirals, fractures, and osteonecrosis in a large international HIV cohort. Clin Infect Dis 2017;64(10):1413–21.

36. Gladman DD, Urowitz MB, Chaudhry-Ahluwalia V, et al. Predictive factors for symptomatic osteonecrosis in patients with systemic lupus erythematosus. J Rheumatol 2001;28:761–5.

37. Kennedy JW, Khan W. Total hip arthroplasty in systemic lupus erythematosus: as systematic review. Int J Rheumatol 2015;2015:475489.

38. Chen D, Cancienne J, Werner B, et al. Is osteonecrosis due to systemic lupus erythematosus associated with increased risk of complications following total hip arthroplasty? Int Orthop 2018; 42:1485–90.

39. Daoud A, Hudson M, Magnus KG, et al. Avascular necrosis of the femoral head after palliative radiotherapy in metastatic prostate cancer: absence of a dose threshold? Cureus 2016;8(3):e521.

40. Pierce TP, Jauregui JJ, Cherian JJ, et al. Imaging evaluation of patients with osteonecrosis of the femoral head. Curr Rev Musculoskelet Med 2015; 8:221–7.

41. Ficat RP. Idiopathic bone necrosis of the femoral head: early diagnosis and treatment. J Bone Joint Surg Br 1985;67-B(1):3–9.

42. Dasa V, Abdel-Nabi, Anders M, et al. F-18 fluoride positron emission tomography of the hip for osteonecrosis. Clin Orthop Relat Res 2008; 466:1081–6.

43. Mont M, Marulanda G, Jones LC, et al. Systematic analysis of classification systems for osteonecrosis of the femoral head. J Bone Joint Surg 2006;88-A-(Supplement 3):16–26.

44. Steinberg ME, Steinberg DR. Classification systems for osteonecrosis: an overview. Orthop Clin N Am 2004;35:273–83.

45. Ha Y, Jung W, Kim J, et al. Prediction of collapse in femoral head osteonecrosis: a modified Kerboul method with use of magnetic resonance images. J Bone Joint Surg 2006;88-A(Supplement 3):35–40.

46. Mont M, Carbon J, Fairbank A. Core decompression versus nonoperative management for osteonecrosis of the hip. Clin Orthop Relat Res 1996; 324:169–78.

47. Mont M, Zywiel M, Marker D, et al. The natural history of untreated osteonecrosis of the femoral head. J Bone Joint Surg 2010;92:2165–70.

48. Lee Y, Ha Y, Cho Y, et al. Does zolendronate prevent femoral head collapse from osteonecrosis? A prospective, randomized, open-label, multicenter study. J Bone Joint Surg 2015;97:1142–8.

49. Agarwala S, Shah S. Ten-year follow-up of avascular necrosis of the femoral head treated with alendronate for 3 years. J Arthroplasty 2011;26(7):1128–34.

50. Yuan HF, Guo CA, Yan ZQ. The use of bisphosphonate in the treatment of osteonecrosis of the femoral head: a meta-analysis of randomized control trials. Osteoporos Int 2016;27:295–9.

51. Li D, Yang Z, Wei Z, et al. Efficacy of bisphosphonates in the treatment of femoral head osteonecrosis: a PRISMA-compliant meta-analysis of animal studies and clinical trials. Sci Rep 2018;8(1):1450.

52. Glueck C, Freiberg R, Wang P. Treatment of osteonecrosis of the hip and knee with enoxaparin. In: Koo K, Mont M, Jones L, editors. Osteonecrosis. Berlin: Springer; 2014. p. 241–7.

53. Cao F, Liu G, Wang W, et al. Combined treatment with an anticoagulant and a vasodilator prevents steroid-associated osteonecrosis of rabbit femoral heads by improving hypercoagulability. Biomed Res Int 2017;2017:1624074.

54. Song Q, Ni J, Jiang H, et al. Sildenafil improves blood perfusion in steroid-induced avascular necrosis of femoral head in rabbits via a protein kinase G-dependent mechanism. Acta Orthop Traumatol Turc 2017;51:298–403.

55. Kandil A, Cui Q. Lipid-lowering agents and their effects on osteonecrosis: pros and cons. In: Koo K, Mont M, Jones L, editors. Osteonecrosis. Berlin: Springer; 2014. p. 255–9.

56. Cui Q, Wang G, Su C, et al. Lovastatin prevents steroid induced adipogenesis and osteonecrosis. Clin Orthop Relat Res 1997;344:8–19.

57. Ajmal M, Matas AJ, Kuskowski M, et al. Does statin use reduce the risk of corticosteroid-related osteonecrosis in renal transplant population? Orthop Clin N Am 2009;40:235–9.

58. Pritchett J. Statin therapy decreases the risk of osteonecrosis in patients receiving steroids. Clin Orthop Relat Res 2001;386:173–8.

59. Wang CJ, Wang FS, Huang CC, et al. Treatment for osteonecrosis of the femoral head: comparison of extracorporeal shock waves with core decompression and bone grafting. J Bone Joint Surg 2005; 87-A(11):2380–7.

60. Al-Jabri T, Tan J, Tong G, et al. The role of electrical stimulation in the management of avascular necrosis of the femoral head in adults: a systematic review. BMC Musculoskelet Disord 2017;18:319.

61. Li W, Ye Z, Wang W, et al. Clinical effect of hyperbaric oxygen therapy in the treatment of femoral

head necrosis: a systematic review and meta-analysis. Orthopade 2017;46:440–6.

62. Pierce TP, Jauregui JJ, Elmallah RK, et al. A current review of core decompression in the treatment of osteonecrosis of the femoral head. Curr Rev Musculoskelet Med 2015;8:228–32.

63. Hernigou P, Beaujean F. Treatment of osteonecrosis with autologous bone marrow grafting. Clin Orthop Relat Res 2002;405:14–23.

64. Houdek MT, Wyles CC, Martin JR, et al. Stem cell treatment for avascular necrosis of the femoral head: current perspectives. Stem Cells Cloning 2014;7:65–70.

65. Larson E, Jones L, Goodman S, et al. Early-stage osteonecrosis of the femoral head: where are we and where are we going in year 2018? Int Orthop 2018;42:1723–8.

66. Houdek MT, Wyles CC, Sierra RJ. Osteonecrosis of the femoral head: treatment with ancillary growth factors. Curr Rev Musculoskelet Med 2015;8:233–9.

67. Houdek MT, Wyles CC, Collins M, et al. Stem cells combined with platelet-rich plasma effectively treat corticosteroid-induced osteonecrosis of the hip: a prospective study. Clin Orthop Relat Res 2018; 476:388–97.

68. Xu S, Zhang L, Jin H, et al. Autologous stem cells combined core decompression for treatment of avascular necrosis of the femoral head: a systematic review. Biomed Res Int 2017;2017:6136205.

69. Millikan PD, Karas V, Wellman S. Treatment of osteonecrosis of the femoral head with vascularized bone grafting. Curr Rev Musculoskelet Med 2015;8: 252–9.

70. Pierce TP, Elmallah RK, Jauregui JJ, et al. A current review of non-vascularized bone grafting in osteonecrosis of the femoral head. Curr Rev Musculoskelet Med 2015;8:240–5.

71. Urbaniak JR, Harvey EJ. Revascularization of the femoral head in osteonecrosis. J Am Acad Orthop Surg 1998;6:44–54.

72. Aldridge JM, Berend KR, Gunneson E, et al. Free vascularized fibular grafting for the treatment of postcollapse osteonecrosis of the femoral head. J Bone Joint Surg 2004;86-A(Supplement 1): 87–101.

73. Cao L, Guo C, Chen J, et al. Free vascularized fibular grafting improves vascularity compared with core decompression in femoral head osteonecrosis: a randomized clinical trial. Clin Orthop Relat Res 2017;475:2230–40.

74. Pierce TP, Elmallah RK, Jauregui JJ, et al. Outcomes of total hip arthroplasty in patients with osteonecrosis of the femoral head—a current review. Curr Rev Musculoskelet Med 2015;8: 246–51.

75. Rinjen W, Lamejin N, Schreurs BW, et al. Total hip arthroplasty after failed treatment for osteonecrosis of the femoral head. Orthop Clin N Am 2009;40: 291–8.

76. Kim SJ, Kang DG, Park SB, et al. Is hemiresurfacing arthroplasty for osteonecrosis of the hip a viable solution? J Arthroplasty 2015;30:987–92.

77. Maguire N, Robertson B, Henman P. Girdlestone procedure for avascular necrosis of the hip in an intravenous drug user. J Surg Case Rep 2014;8 [pii:rju039].

78. Kamath AF, McGraw MH, Israelite CL. Surgical management of osteonecrosis of the femoral head in patients with sickle cell disease. World J Orthop 2015;6(10):776–82.

79. Kim-Orden M, Barret K, Khatod M. Algorithm for treatment of hip and knee osteonecrosis: review and Presentation of three examples cases. J Rheum Dis Treat 2017;3:053.

Cost-Effectiveness of Dual Mobility and a Value-Based Algorithm of Utilization

Hayeem L. Rudy, BA[a], Jorge A. Padilla, MD[a],
Jonathan A. Gabor, BS[a], Richard Iorio, MD[b],
Ran Schwarzkopf, MD, MSc[a], Jonathan Vigdorchik, MD[a],*

KEYWORDS

- Dual mobility cups • Unconstrained tripolar implant • Cost-effectiveness • Cost-analysis
- Economic analysis • Total hip arthroplasty

KEY POINTS

- Despite the well-documented clinical outcomes of total hip arthroplasty (THA), hip dislocation secondary to instability and the financial burden associated with treatment efforts remain disconcerting.
- Dual mobility (DM) bearings effectively reduce the rate of prosthetic hip dislocation and may, therefore, be a cost-effective alternative for THA in patients with increased risk of dislocation.
- In terms of implant failure, to be cost-effective, novel medical devices such as DM systems must reduce the revision surgery rate by 10% to 20%.
- There is a paucity of literature evaluating the long-term survivorship and clinical outcomes of modern DM systems that must be assessed before decisions are made regarding its use for routine primary THA in the general population.
- Novel DM systems may effectively reduce the overall health care expenditures associated with THA, if the price-difference between these and the conventional prostheses remains below $1023.

INTRODUCTION

Total joint arthroplasty (TJA) is widely considered to be the paradigmatic example of successful orthopedic surgery in the last 50 years due to the reliability with which it restores function and alleviates pain.[1] Accordingly, the rates at which these operations are being performed have been steadily increasing, such that by 2030, it is projected that more than half of a million total hip arthroplasties (THAs) will be performed.[2] Currently, TJA accounts for more Medicare spending than any other single inpatient medical procedure, exceeding $9 billion of the Medicare budget annually, and is expected to exceed $50 billion by 2030.[3] Despite the relatively exceptional outcomes of THA, hip dislocation remains a major concern due to the high frequency of occurrence and the increased financial burden it places on the US health care system.

Hip dislocation secondary to instability is a frequent and significant complication following THA that has extensive clinical and economic implications. Dislocation is the single most common reason for all-component revision THA and for isolated acetabular component revision.[4] Approximately one-third of hip dislocations in conventional implants fail closed-reduction and

Disclosure Statement: The authors have not received any financial support related to the production of this article.
[a] Department of Orthopedic Surgery, NYU Langone Orthopedic Hospital, NYU Langone Health, 301 East 17th Street, New York, NY 10003, USA; [b] Department of Orthopaedic Surgery, Brigham and Women's Hospital, Harvard Medical School, 60 Fenwood Road, Boston, MA 02115, USA
* Corresponding author. NYU Langone Orthopedic Hospital, NYU Langone Health, Hospital for Joint Diseases, 301 East 17th Street, New York, NY 10003.
E-mail address: jvigdorchik@gmail.com

non-surgical efforts and must subsequently undergo surgical revision intervention.[5,6] The economic burden of these revision surgeries and for closed-reduction attempts following dislocation are significant.[6] Consequently, much attention has been paid to understanding the variables that influence the risk of dislocation. Alongside advances in surgical techniques, improvement in implant design have been critical to reducing the risk of dislocation by increasing the femoral neck length and offset, maximizing femoral head size in relation to the femoral neck, and improving articulation design.[7,8]

The dual mobility (DM) cup, also known as an unconstrained tripolar implant, proposed by Bousquet in 1974, is one such design that features 2 articulations, the first between the femoral head implant and an inner polyethylene cup, and the second between the polyethylene cup and an outer metal acetabular shell.[9] This design increases range of motion, enlarges the effective size of the femoral head relative to the femoral neck, and minimizes prosthesis neck impingement and head jump distance, ultimately reducing the risk of dislocation. Following the 2009 US Food and Drug Administration regulatory approval of this articulation in North America, DM cups are now widely implemented in patients who are predisposed to developing postoperative instability. The current literature reporting on the efficacy of the designs suggests that, indeed, DM cups are effective at reducing the risk of instability-related complications.[10,11] Despite the advantages offered by DM systems, it is imperative that the additional clinical benefits be weighed against the considerable economic costs associated with these implants. Furthermore, it is critical that the idiosyncratic failure mechanisms of DM cups, such as intraprosthetic dislocation (IPD), be appropriately scrutinized because they may decrease long-term survivorship and increase costs associated to THA.[12]

As competition for a limited pool of health care resources increases, it is critical that health care decision-makers allocate resources efficiently and maximize value to society. This article reviews the literature regarding the cost-effectiveness of DM systems as an alternative to standard articulations.

MATERIALS AND METHODS

A comprehensive, retrospective review of literature analyzing the current peer-reviewed data available on the electronic PubMed database was undertaken on July 10, 2018. The literature search was performed to identify potentially relevant studies for inclusion in this article that were focused primarily on the cost-effectiveness of DM cups use in THA. The literature search and screening were performed by 2 independent review authors. To include the most suitable and representative literature, an initial query was primed in the PubMed database for the following terms: dual mobility, tripolar implants, cost-effectiveness, cost-analysis, or economic analysis. The primary search yielded 228 articles. Studies were eligible for inclusion if they were written in the English language, discussed or compared the cost-effectiveness of THA with the DM cup, and were published from January 1995 through June 2018. The titles and abstracts of the initial search results were screened for the previously mentioned terms and content relevance. Review articles, editorials, descriptive discussions, and case reports were excluded from this study. The full-text of the retained titles and abstracts was then further scrutinized in detail to further assess eligibility. Additionally, references of the retrieved articles were correspondingly screened for further inclusion of relevant literature. Only those articles that met the aforementioned criteria were included in the present literature review.

RESULTS

The primary literature search identified a total of 239 potentially eligible articles (**Fig. 1**). A total of 220 were discarded following the initial screening of the title and abstract due to failing to fulfill the criteria or to fall within the scope of this review. Nineteen studies met the inclusion criteria and were deemed relevant for the literature review. An additional 5 articles were extracted from the references of the previously retained articles. Therefore, a total of 24 were included in the final literature review.

Factors Influencing Cost-Effectiveness of New Total Hip Arthroplasty Implant Technology

In discussing the cost-effectiveness of DM cups versus traditional articulations, it is necessary to identify the primary variables that determine the cost-effectiveness of the alternative prosthesis. Faulkner and colleagues[13] performed an extensive cost-effectiveness analysis of data derived from the British National Health Service and found that there were only 3 primary variables that determined the cost-effectiveness of a prosthesis. These variables were

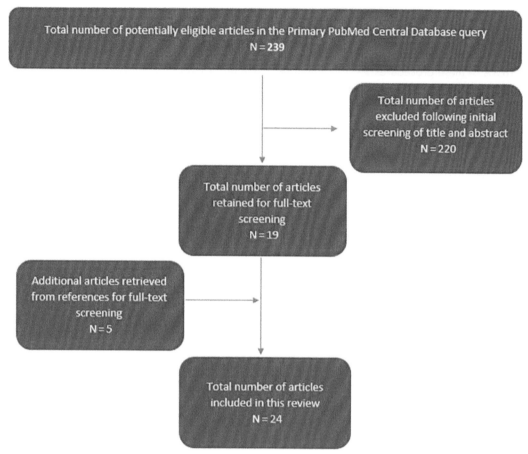

Fig. 1. Flow diagram illustrating the selection process of potentially eligible articles for inclusion in the present review of literature.

1. Implant cost
2. Hospital cost
3. Revision rate.[13]

In this review, Faulkner and colleagues[13] demonstrated a new prosthesis with a 0% revision rate would only be cost-effective if the cost of the implant was equivalent to or less than double the cost of a cemented Charnley prosthesis.

Another extensive review by Fitzpatrick and colleagues[14] determined that for new prosthesis priced at 300% of a standard Charnley prosthesis at the time of the study, a reduction in revision rates between 35% and 44% in patients aged 50 to 70 years, and between 21% and 27% in patients aged younger than 50 years, would be required. For a new prosthesis at 150% the cost of the standard implant, a 9% to 12% improvement in revision rates in patients aged 50 to 70 years, and a 6% to 7% improvement in patients aged 50 years or younger would be required for it to be cost-effective.[14]

Similarly, Gillespie and colleagues[15] analyzed data from the Swedish Joint Registry and determined that in a young (<50 years) active THA recipient, an implant that offered a 15% reduction in the risk of revision surgery at 15 years postoperatively could be sold for 2 to 2.5 times the cost of a Charnley prosthesis and remain cost-effective. The same investigators reported that the cost-effectiveness of a newer technology implant was reduced significantly in older patients of either gender.

Finally, Bozic and colleagues[16] performed a cost-effective analysis to evaluate the reduction in revision rate that would be necessary for a newer technology prosthesis with an incremental cost of $2000 in 2006 to be cost-effective and determined this value to be a 19% reduction in 20-year revision rate. They also concluded that such prosthesis would not be cost-effective in patients older than the age of 75 years.[16]

Economic Impact of Dislocation
Dislocation rates are critical to determining the cost-effectiveness of a given prosthesis because

of the costs associated with both closed and open reduction attempts, as well as revision surgery. Dislocation is currently the most common reason for revision THA, accounting for 22.5% to 26.3% of these procedures.[4,17] The literature suggests that approximately one-third of patients with dislocation ultimately require revision surgery.[4,6]

Sanchez-Sotelo and colleagues[6] reported on the total hospital cost of dislocation at a single institution after primary THA. In this study, all of 99 patients who experienced dislocation were treated with at least 1 attempt at closed reduction with or without subsequent revision surgery. Each attempted closed reduction represented 19% of the total hospital cost for an uncomplicated primary THA at the same hospital in 2003. Adjusting for inflation, total cost of primary THA was approximately $16,759. Therefore, the cost of each closed reduction attempt after THA was an additional $3184. The average total hospital cost for revision surgery following dislocation was 148% of the cost of an uncomplicated THA. Adjusted for inflation, the total average hospital cost of 1 or more closed reductions and the subsequent revision surgery was $27,987.[6]

In 2009, Bozic and colleagues[4] reviewed the costs associated with revision THA in a cohort of more than 50,000 patients from the Nationwide Inpatient Sample Database. They reported an average total charge of $54,553 for revision THA. The most common reason for revision THA in the cohort was instability and dislocation. This study included a variety of revision THA procedures ranging from head and liner exchange to all-component revision. Almost all revisions in this study were all-component revision, and the range of costs for procedures of any type was $42,245 to $69,380.[4]

Probability of Dislocation in Dual Mobility Systems Versus Traditional Articulation Systems

The incidence of dislocation in THA with non-DM implants is time-dependent. The most cited literature reports a cumulative risk of first-time dislocation of 1% at 1 month, 1.9% at 1 year, and then a constant additional 1% for every 5 years, such that the cumulative risk at 25 years postoperatively is roughly 7%. Dislocation rates may be substantially higher in patients who present with risk factors that predispose to instability, such as a history of avascular necrosis, inflammatory arthritis, dementia, lower socioeconomic status, and discharge to skilled nursing facility.[18] Large-scale studies in the literature have demonstrated a 10% cumulative dislocation rate in patients undergoing primary THA for femoral neck fracture at 10 years postoperatively.[19] Similarly, large studies have demonstrated a long-term cumulative dislocation rate of 20% in patients older than 80 years old.[20]

Vigdorchik and colleagues[21] conducted the largest study examining clinical outcomes following the use of DM implants. Their study analyzed 485 hips and reported on outcomes within 2 years postoperatively. They reported zero large articulation dislocations and zero IPDs. A retrospective, matched, comparative analysis published by Rowan and colleagues[22] evaluated the short-term outcomes of DM versus traditional-bearing cohorts at a single institution in a younger patient population. The investigators matched 136 subjects who underwent THA with highly cross-linked polyethylene DM with a cohort of 136 patients who received a fixed-bearing. Their comparative analysis found 0% dislocation in the DM cohort and 5.1% in the fixed-bearing cohort with an average follow-up of 3.2 and 3.4 years, respectively. Boyer and colleagues[23] conducted the longest follow-up study of DM components in the literature. They found zero dislocations in 240 hips over 22 years.

Unlike traditional articulations, DM implants are susceptible to idiosyncratic failure mechanisms. One important failure mechanism is IPD, in which the femoral head dislocates from the inner polyethylene cup. Early generations of DM cups reported a relatively high 3% to 5% IPD rate.[10,24,25] However, subsequent DM designs incorporated highly cross-linked polyethylene inner cups that reinforced the retentive mechanism acting on the femoral head and this ultimately led to a greater than 10-fold reduction in IPD.[25] There is a paucity of data on long-term IPD rates in newer DM designs. In contrast to traditional implants, in DM prosthesis, IPD cannot be reduced nonoperatively. Consequently, they always require DM bearing revision and may potentially require shell revision, leading to an increase in total expenditures per episode of care.[26,27]

Implant Cost of Dual Mobility Systems Versus Traditional Articulation Systems

Differences in implant cost play a critical role in determining the cost-effectiveness of new implant designs. As previously discussed, several studies have reported that new implant technologies are typically cost-effective when their implant costs do not exceed between 1.2 and 2.0 times the cost of the traditional implant, and when they successfully reduce the revision surgery rate by 15% to 20% for 15 to 20 years postoperatively.[4,13–15]

DM and conventional implants typically have equally priced chromium-cobalt femoral heads and femoral stems. According to *Orthopedic Network News* (Mendenhall Associates, Inc, Ann Arbor, Michigan, USA),[28] which provides current financial information on the US hip and knee implant market, the average selling price of the conventional and DM systems are as follows:

- Classic: metal-on-poly construct ($1766), trident cup ($888), polyethylene liner ($909)
- DM: metal-on-mobile bearing polyethylene construct ($2766), trident cup ($888), large polyethylene ball insert ($909).

The $1000 price difference represents the incremental expenditures associated with using a DM cup in comparison with the conventional system.

Previously, cost-containment efforts have successfully reduced the total health care expenditures for THA by controlling the cost of hospital supplies and orthopedic devices, particularly implant cost. In 2012, the New York University Langone Medical Center an urban, academic, orthopedic specialty hospital, now NYU Langone Health, effectively reduced the average implant cost per case by 22% to 33% following the implementation of a price ceiling implant cost-control protocol.[29] Similarly, the Lahey Clinic implemented a cost-containment program focused primarily on reducing the total cost of their implants.[30] They successfully reduced implant cost by 23%. Following these successful implant cost negotiations, future patient-centered, value-based programs will be crucial for effectively maintaining the cost of novel articulations such as the DM cup.

DISCUSSION

The frequency and cost of hip dislocation following THA remains a major concern in orthopedics, which imposes a serious economic burden on the US health care system. Despite advancements in prosthesis design and surgical technique, hip dislocation still remains a common and costly complication.[4,26] Since the relatively recent introduction of modern DM systems, early short-term clinical studies investigating their efficacy have demonstrated low rates of dislocation.[21,23] However, despite these clinical improvements, the question of whether

DM components are cost-effective in both the general population and in specific subpopulations in the United States remains unanswered.

In the absence of sufficient published data, uncertainty regarding the appropriate use of DM components requires evaluation of the advantages and disadvantages of this intervention in comparison to conventional THA systems. Recently, Barlow and colleagues[31] performed a cost-effective analysis using a Markov model to investigate the cost-effectiveness of DM components versus a conventional THA system. Their study found the DM systems failed to be cost-effective when the cost of the implant exceeds that of the traditional system by $1023. In the current study, analysis of the difference between the average sale price between the DM and traditional systems was $1,000, which borders on this cost threshold. Barlow and colleagues[31] also found that DM components failed to be cost-effective when the annualized incremental probability (AIP) of IPD, large articulation dislocation, or failure from unforeseen mechanisms exceeded 0.49%, 0.29%, or 0.29%, respectively. Although the most cited and highly powered studies of modern DM designs report the AIP of intraprosthetic dislocation to fall short of this threshold, there is a paucity of long-term data on modern DM designs. Moreover, several studies reporting at least 15 years of follow-up in hips with early DM designs have reported AIP rates of IPD that border on and exceed those thresholds (range of AIP: 0.042%–0.47%).[12,32] The DM designs in these studies included conventional polyethylene versus the highly cross-linked polyethylene in modern designs that offers a more robust retentive mechanism and prevents femoral head dislocation from the polyethylene liner. Nonetheless, long-term studies are needed to determine the rate of IPD in these novel designs because this will have a significant impact on the cost-effectiveness of these implants.

Epinette and colleagues[33] similarly described their results with the use of Markov modeling to assess the cost-effectiveness of DM components compared with fixed-bearing components for patients undergoing THA in France. In their sensitivity analysis, they found that DM components resulted in greater cost-saving than fixed-bearing components under all hypothesis and generated maximum cost-savings in excess of €100 million annually.

Whether the application of DM systems for primary THA adds value in healthy patients who do not have clinical predisposition to dislocate remains unknown. However, it is probable that this paradigm changes in patients who are at high risk of dislocation. In this setting, outcomes, including rates of dislocation, revision surgery, and ongoing care needs associated with dislocation, would be substantially improved for high-risk patients receiving a DM implant. Concurrently, health care expenditures associated with the utilization of a DM system in such patients would be reduced when compared with the total costs of using traditional implants in the same patient. Therefore, the creation of increased value is achievable ensuing the utilization of DM when selection for patients at greater risk of dislocation is implemented.

To improve the value of DM systems, health care institutions may also benefit from the implementation of screening protocols intended to identify patients at risk of developing instability and dislocation. Such protocols might identify critical variables that increase the risk of dislocation. In addition to known risk factors for dislocation, such as gender and increased age, it would be important for screening protocols to incorporate strong but less traditional risk factors. One risk factor that has been incorporated in screening protocols at New York University, Langone Orthopedic Hospital, is a history of lumbar-pelvic fusion surgery, which has been demonstrated to increase the rate of prosthetic hip dislocation more than 7-fold within 12 months postoperatively.[34–36]

The present study identified an implant cost difference of $1000 between DM and conventional systems. It is important to note that price variability of implants is dynamic and subject not only to change with inflation but also other market forces such as geographic location.[37] There is evidence in the literature that suggests the cost difference between novel and traditional implants on the market decreases over time. Moreover, implant price negotiation by health institutions with vendors has also been shown to have a significant impact on the average sale price of implants. Bosco and colleagues[29] and Healy and colleagues[30] demonstrated that price negotiations via a standardized price initiative are a feasible method of reducing the price implants. These dynamic factors must also be considered when comparing DM versus traditional systems and should be interpreted in the context of a given practice setting (ie, large health care institution vs private practice setting).

SUMMARY

Based on the current data, DM systems may be an important component for the future success of value-based THA. In comparison to conventional implants, the benefits of DM systems, particularly decreased postoperative hip instability, are well-documented. Novel DM systems are more likely to be cost-effective if the incremental expenditure of the system does not exceed the price of conventional systems by approximately $1023. Furthermore, for DM to be cost-effective, the implant failure and the subsequent need for revision surgery rate should be 10% to 20% less than the rate of conventional implant systems. There is a paucity of literature evaluating the long-term rates of idiosyncratic failure mechanisms in modern DM systems, which may further affect the cost-effectiveness of this implant. Accordingly, before incorporating DM cup for routine primary THA in the general population, future clinical studies are necessary to assess the long-term clinical outcomes of novel DM systems.

REFERENCES

1. Learmonth ID, Young C, Rorabeck C. The operation of the century: total hip replacement. Lancet 2007;370(9597):1508–19.
2. Kurtz S, Ong K, Lau E, et al. Projections of primary and revision hip and knee arthroplasty in the United States from 2005 to 2030. J Bone Joint Surg Am 2007;89(4):780–5.
3. Stambough JB, Nunley RM, Curry MC, et al. Rapid recovery protocols for primary total hip arthroplasty can safely reduce length of stay without increasing readmissions. J Arthroplasty 2015;30(4):521–6.
4. Bozic KJ, Kurtz SM, Lau E, et al. The epidemiology of revision total hip arthroplasty in the United States. J Bone Joint Surg Am 2009;91(1):128–33.
5. Berry DJ, von Knoch M, Schleck CD, et al. The cumulative long-term risk of dislocation after primary Charnley total hip arthroplasty. J Bone Joint Surg Am 2004;86-A(1):9–14. Available at: http://www.ncbi.nlm.nih.gov/pubmed/14711939. Accessed July 24, 2018.
6. Sanchez-Sotelo J, Haidukewych GJ, Boberg CJ. Hospital cost of dislocation after primary total hip arthroplasty. 2006. Available at: https://insights.ovid.com/pubmed?pmid=16452739. Accessed July 24, 2018.
7. Callaghan JJ, O'Rourke MR, Goetz DD, et al. Use of a constrained tripolar acetabular liner to treat intraoperative instability and postoperative dislocation after total hip arthroplasty: a review of our experience. Clin Orthop Relat Res 2004;429:117–23. Available at: http://www.ncbi.nlm.nih.gov/pubmed/15577475. Accessed July 26, 2018.

8. Daly PJ, Morrey BF. Operative correction of an unstable total hip arthroplasty. J Bone Joint Surg Am 1992; 74(9):1334–43. Available at: http://www.ncbi.nlm.nih.gov/pubmed/1429788. Accessed July 26, 2018.

9. Grazioli A, Ek ETH, Rüdiger HA. Biomechanical concept and clinical outcome of dual mobility cups. Int Orthop 2012;36(12):2411–8.

10. Massin P, Orain V, Philippot R, et al. Fixation failures of dual mobility cups a mid-term study of 2601 hip replacements clinical orthopaedics and related research ® a publication of the association of bone and joint surgeons®. Clin Orthop Relat Res 2012;470:1932–40.

11. Luthra JS, Al Riyami A, Allami MK. Dual mobility total hip replacement in a high risk population. SICOT J 2016;2:43.

12. Banka TR, Ast MP, Parks ML. Early intraprosthetic dislocation in a revision dual-mobility hip prosthesis. Orthopedics 2014;37(4):e395–7.

13. Faulkner A, Kennedy LG, Baxter K, et al. Effectiveness of hip prostheses in primary total hip replacement: a critical review of evidence and an economic model. Health Technol Assess 1998;2(6):1–133. Available at: http://www.ncbi.nlm.nih.gov/pubmed/9728294. Accessed July 26, 2018.

14. Fitzpatrick R, Shortall E, Sculpher M, et al. Primary total hip replacement surgery: a systematic review of outcomes and modelling of cost-effectiveness associated with different prostheses. Health Technol Assess 1998;2(20):1–64. Available at: http://www.ncbi.nlm.nih.gov/pubmed/10103353. Accessed July 26, 2018.

15. Gillespie WJ, Pekarsky B, O'Connell DL. Evaluation of new technologies for total hip replacement. Economic modelling and clinical trials. J Bone Joint Surg Br 1995;77(4):528–33. Available at: http://www.ncbi.nlm.nih.gov/pubmed/7615594. Accessed July 26, 2018.

16. Bozic KJ, Morshed S, Silverstein MD, et al. Use of cost-effectiveness analysis to evaluate new technologies in orthopaedics: the case of alternative bearing surfaces in total hip arthroplasty. J Bone Joint Surg Am 2006;88(4):706–14.

17. Fourth AJRR annual report on hip and knee arthroplasty data. Available at: http://www.ajrr.net/images/annual_reports/AJRR-2017-Annual-Report—Final.pdf. Accessed July 24, 2018.

18. Gausden EB, Parhar HS, Popper JE, et al. Risk factors for early dislocation following primary elective total hip arthroplasty. J Arthroplasty 2018;33(5):1567–71.e2.

19. Tarasevicius S, Jermolajevas V, Tarasevicius R, et al. Total hip replacement for the treatment of femoral neck fractures. Long-term results. Medicina (Kaunas) 2005;41(6):465–9.

20. Levy RN, Levy CM, Snyder J, et al. Outcome and long-term results following total hip replacement in elderly patients. Clin Orthop Relat Res 1995;(316):25–30. Available at: http://www.ncbi.nlm.nih.gov/pubmed/7634714. Accessed July 25, 2018.

21. Vigdorchik JM, D'Apuzzo MR, Markel DC, et al. Lack of early dislocation following total hip arthroplasty with a new dual mobility acetabular design. Hip Int 2015;25(1):34–8.

22. Rowan FE, Salvatore AJ, Lange JK, et al. Dual-mobility vs fixed-bearing total hip arthroplasty in patients under 55 years of age: a single-institution, matched-cohort analysis. J Arthroplasty 2017;32(10):3076–81.

23. Boyer B, Philippot R, Geringer J. Primary total hip arthroplasty with dual mobility socket to prevent dislocation: a 22-year follow-up of 240 hips. Int Orthop 2012;36(3):511–8.

24. Philippot R, Camilleri JP, Boyer B, et al. The use of a dual-articulation acetabular cup system to prevent dislocation after primary total hip arthroplasty: analysis of 384 cases at a mean follow-up of 15 years. Int Orthop 2009;33(4):927–32.

25. Philippot R, Boyer B, Farizon F. Intraprosthetic dislocation: a specific complication of the dual-mobility system. Clin Orthop Relat Res 2013; 471(3):965–70.

26. Waddell BS, De Martino I, Sculco T, et al. Total hip arthroplasty dislocations are more complex than they appear: a case report of intraprosthetic dislocation of an anatomic dual-mobility implant after closed reduction. Available at: https://search-proquest-com.ezproxy.med.nyu.edu/docview/1795655347/fulltextPDF/B8355CDF9D904B43PQ/1?accountid=12768. Accessed July 25, 2018.

27. De Martino I, D'Apolito R, Waddell BS, et al. Early intraprosthetic dislocation in dual-mobility implants: a systematic review. Arthroplast Today 2017;3(3):197–202.

28. 2016 Hip and knee implant review. Orthopedic network news. Available at: www.orthopedicnetworknews.com. Accessed July 31, 2018.

29. Bosco JA, Alvarado CM, Slover JD, et al. Decreasing total joint implant costs and physician specific cost variation through negotiation. J Arthroplasty 2014;29(4):678–80.

30. Healy WL, Iorio R, Lemos MJ, et al. Single price/case price purchasing in orthopaedic surgery: experience at the Lahey Clinic. J Bone Joint Surg Am 2000;82(5):607–12.

31. Barlow BT, Mclawhorn AS, Westrich GH. The cost-effectiveness of dual mobility implants for primary total hip arthroplasty: a computer-based cost-utility model. J Bone Joint Surg Am 2017;99(9):768–77.

32. Guyen O, Chen QS, Bejui-Hugues J, et al. Unconstrained tripolar hip implants: effect on hip stability. Clin Orthop Relat Res 2007;455:202–8.

33. Epinette J-A, Lafuma A, Robert J, et al. Cost-effectiveness model comparing dual-mobility to fixed-bearing designs for total hip replacement in France. Orthop Traumatol Surg Res 2016;102(2):143–8.

34. Buckland AJ, Puvanesarajah V, Vigdorchik J, et al. Dislocation of a primary total hip arthroplasty is more common in patients with a lumbar spinal fusion. Bone Joint J 2017;99-B(5):585–91.

35. Perfetti DC, Schwarzkopf R, Buckland AJ, et al. Prosthetic Dislocation and Revision After Primary Total Hip Arthroplasty in Lumbar Fusion Patients: A Propensity Score Matched-Pair Analysis. J Arthroplasty 2017. https://doi.org/10.1016/j.arth.2016.11.029.

36. Buckland AJ, Vigdorchik J, Schwab FJ, et al. Acetabular anteversion changes due to spinal deformity correction: bridging the gap between hip and spine surgeons. J Bone Joint Surg Am 2015;97(23):1913–20.

37. Robinson JC, Pozen A, Tseng S, et al. Variability in costs associated with total hip and knee replacement implants. J Bone Jt Surg - Ser A 2012. https://doi.org/10.2106/JBJS.K.00355.

Trauma

Locked Plating and Advanced Augmentation Techniques in Osteoporotic Fractures

Graham J. DeKeyser, MD, Patrick J. Kellam, MD,
Justin M. Haller, MD*

KEYWORDS

- Osteoporosis • Locked plate • Fragility fracture • Elderly • Endosteal replacement

KEY POINTS

- Osteoporotic fractures represent unique fixation challenges related to decreased bone mineral density and higher rates of screw pullout.
- Locked plating creates a fixed-angle construct with greater resistance to failure in osteoporotic bone with thin cortices.
- Osteoporotic fractures can be supplemented with endosteal replacement (nail or fibula allograft) or an additional plate to provide greater stability to the overall construct.
- Polymethyl methacrylate or calcium-derived bone cements can strengthen screw purchase and limit screw pullout or they can be used to resist compressive failure.

INTRODUCTION

In 2002, the National Osteoporosis Foundation estimated that around 10 million adults older than 50 years suffered from osteoporosis in the United States.[1] Wright and colleagues[2] expanded on this report and predicted that by 2020, 11.9 million people, in the same population range as the 2002 report, would be suffering from osteoporosis.

Fragility fractures are expected to continue to increase and have been predicted to exceed 3 million incident fractures by the year 2025.[3] Furthermore, these fractures are expected to cost the United States more than 25 billion dollars in care expenses.[3] Hip fractures are the costliest of these fractures, amassing 72% of all costs for only 14% of the total volume of fractures. Although these fractures are associated with significant cost, it is their poor outcomes that impart a large societal burden. The 1-year mortality following elderly hip fracture is routinely reported to be around 25%.[4,5] Moreover, rates of postoperative nursing facility placement have been reported up to 60%.[3,5–7] As such, caring for osteoporotic fractures is and will continue to be a large part of the orthopedic surgeon's practice.

Pathophysiology of Osteoporosis

Although there are numerous secondary causes of osteoporosis, most of the cases are thought to be age related. Trabecular bone loss is typically the initial finding. Modulated mostly by estrogen, this trabecular thinning is a constellation of resorption from trabecular bone, including a decrease in the number of trabecular plates.[8–11] Although dual-energy x-ray absorptiometry

Disclosure Statement: The authors have no disclosures of direct financial interest in this subject matter or materials discussed within this article.
University of Utah, Department of Orthopaedics, Orthopaedic Center, 590 Wakara Way, Salt Lake City, UT 84108, USA
* Corresponding author.
E-mail address: Justin.haller@hsc.utah.edu

scans remain the standard for the diagnosis of osteoporosis, this may not correlate with hip fractures.[12,13] Furthermore, recent research has focused on the use of quantitative computed tomography for measuring bone mineral density (BMD). Riggs and colleagues[14] looked at the numerous measurements of different sites of the human skeleton throughout the aging process. They found that both men and women lose cortical area, trabecular volumetric BMD (vBMD), and cortical vBMD. However, women tend to have a larger percentage of loss than men. These findings have been corroborated in other studies using similar techniques.[15,16]

Screw Mechanics and the Effect of Osteoporosis

The most important aspects of a screw design include the outer diameter, core diameter, and pitch. For nonlocking screws, it is important to have a screw with enough bony purchase, a large enough core diameter to prevent shear stresses, and a large enough pitch to insert in a reasonable amount of time.[17,18] Nonlocking plate and screw constructs rely on adequate frictional forces between the plate and bone in order to avoid failure. These plates counter the axial or compressive forces via the shear force at the plate-bone interface. This force is equal to the force normal to the plate multiplied by the plate-bone coefficient of friction. Importantly, the force normal to the plate is a function of the axial force applied to the plate by the torque of the screws that fix the plate to the bone.[17]

Osteoporosis, as described previously, leads to a state of decreased BMD, which results in weaker mechanical properties of the bone. This results in a higher rate of fractures in this population and unique challenges in fracture fixation.[19] BMD has a direct relationship with screw purchase and pullout strength. Traditional plate-and-screw constructs demonstrate an unacceptably high rate of failure in osteoporotic fracture fixation.[20] Cancellous screws that have an increased pitch and outer diameter can aid in fixation in osteoporotic and metaphyseal bone. However, human and animal models have shown that the advantages of cancellous screws are no longer valid below a threshold BMD of 0.4 g/cm^3.[21]

Therefore, osteoporotic bone may not have sufficient mechanical properties to resist the shear forces generated by advancing screw threads. Nonlocking 3.5 mm cortical screws are ideally inserted with approximately 3 to 5 Nm of torque.[22] Osteoporotic models have demonstrated varying levels of maximum torque insertion of conventional screws to be between approximately 1.5 N and 3 N.[23,24] In cadaveric femur models, 3 N of screw torque in standard plates with 3.5 cortical screws began to see motion at the bone-plate interface with as little as 500 N loads.[24] Assuming the human tibia experiences loads up to 4.7 times bodyweight, a patient who weighs 180 pounds would place greater than 500 N force on the tibia with just 15% weight bearing.[25]

If the friction between the bone and plate is overcome, the fixation becomes dependent on the stiffness of single screws. More specifically, the strength of the construct to resist compression becomes equal to the axial stiffness of the single screws farthest from the fracture site depending on where the load is initiated.[26] In a standard plate construct, the axial stiffness depends on the torque between the screw and near cortex, which can be very weak in osteoporotic bone. This can lead to screw loosening and pullout with bone failure and local resorption.[17]

LOCKING PLATES

The first locking type device in orthopedics was the ZESPOL locking fixator. This device used a special designed washer to lock the screw into the plate.[27] Locked plate constructs create a single-beam construct by controlling the axial orientation of the screw as it threads into the plate. Essentially, locked plates function as an external fixator device that is internally located and much closer to the bone. The proximity to the bone and fracture makes these constructs extremely rigid.[28] Typical locking plate indications include osteoporotic bone and short segment articular fractures.

Locking screws do not rely on the friction between the screw head and the plate for fixation. Rather, they are fixed-angle devices that function more as bolts than as screws. They function by transferring the load that the plate sees across all of the screws of the plate directly to the near cortex. As such, this necessitates the larger core diameter of a locking screw to resident the shear stresses it withstands.[28] Because all screws are threaded into the plate at fixed angles and there is no motion between the plate and the screw, they must pull out as a unit and overcome the bone-screw interface at all screws.[26,29,30] This situation is often preferred in osteoporotic bone where plate-to-bone compression is limited by the decreased BMD and thinner cortices. Furthermore, the fixed-angle nature of the locked plate beam construct allows them stronger resistance to cantilever bending.[26]

The single beam construct is 4 times stronger than load-sharing constructs.[31] In large part, this is because locked plates convert shear stress at the bone-plate interface to compressive stress and bone has much higher resistance to compressive forces.[26] Another, advantage of locked plates is that they can preserve periosteal blood supply if applied correctly. Traditional plates rely on the friction between bone and plate for stability, whereas locked plate constructs do not. Theoretically, this preservation of periosteal blood supply creates an environment more conducive to healing.[32]

Proximal Humerus

Most of the proximal humerus fractures can be treated nonoperatively. Significant challenges exist in treatment of operative osteoporotic proximal humerus fractures. Locked plates have had improved results over nonlocking constructs.[33,34] Kralinger and colleagues[35] reviewed 150 surgically treated proximally humerus fractures with locked plates and found no correlation between fixation failure and BMD. However, failure of fixation and screw cutout rates have been reported to happen in 29% of elderly 3-part proximal humerus fractures.[36] In 2009, Südkamp prospectively evaluated 187 patients with proximal humerus fractures treated with locked plate fixation. They noted good overall functional outcomes but had a significant number of complications, most commonly humeral head screw perforation (14%).[37] A systematic review of proximal humerus fractures treated with locked plates found an overall reoperation rate of 13.7% in 791 patients. The review concludes that this high failure and reoperation rate may be due to very rigid constructs in the setting of osteoporotic bone, which often lacks medial calcar support.[38] In proximal humerus fractures with medial calcar comminution, fibula strut allograft supplementation may offer additional stability to the overall construct and help prevent varus collapse.[39] Fixation of osteoporotic fractures of the proximal humerus is certainly an arena where there is need for improved fixation strategies and future research.

Distal Radius

Distal radius fractures are the most common fractures in the appendicular skeleton and account for 18% of fracture incidence in the elderly.[19,40] Again, many of these injuries can be treated nonoperatively with adequate reduction. Volar locking plate fixation of these injuries

has shown improved results compared with other methods of fixation and allow for early range of motion.[41–43] Overall, operative treatment of these injuries with volar locked plates has shown excellent clinical outcomes.[44,45] However, the most recent AAOS practice guidelines could not recommend for or against locked plating and stated that the current evidence regarding locked plating versus percutaneous pinning was "inconclusive."[46]

Distal Femur

Lateral locking plates are commonly used for distal femur fractures, particularly in osteoporotic bone. Locked plating of distal femur fractures has demonstrated excellent union rates and acceptable complication rates compared with other fixation methods.[47] Kregor and colleagues[48] reported on their results of AO type 33 and combined type 33/32 fractures of the distal femur fixed with Less Invasive Stabilization System (LISS). Of 103 fractures, 93% went on to union without secondary procedure and all fractures healed after a secondary procedure including bone grafting. They reported low complication rates including no cases of varus collapse. Despite these promising early results, others found higher nonunion rates in distal femur fractures treated with locked plates. Ricci and colleagues[49] reviewed 335 such cases and found a nonunion rate of 19%. They identified increased body mass index, open fracture, smoking, and shorter plate length as risk factors for plate failure.

Ankle Fractures

Similar to other areas of the body, the incidence of osteoporotic ankle fractures is increasing.[50] The ankle offers a unique opportunity for surgeons to increase screw purchase by placing screws into the tibia and achieving quadcortical fixation (**Fig. 1**). The extra cortical fixation can allow surgeons to avoid locked plates for the fibula.[51] In addition, placing an intramedullary Steinmann pin is another technical trick to getting metallic interference and improving screw purchase. However, if these techniques fail to offer improved screw purchase, fibular locked plating is a reliable option.

AUGMENTATION TECHNIQUES
Dual Plating

One augmentation strategy for osteoporotic fractures is the use of dual plating (**Fig. 2**). This technique has been described for fractures of the distal femur, proximal tibia, and distal humerus among others. The purpose of dual

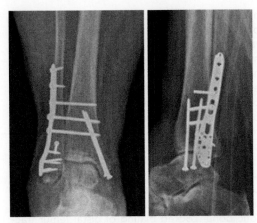

Fig. 1. A 73-year-old man with postoperative antero-posterior (AP) and lateral ankle views demonstrating quad-cortical screw fixation combined with lateral fibular locking plate.

plating is to achieve balanced fixation while not completely relying on the screws of a single construct.

Although a lateral locking plate or retrograde intramedullary nail are commonly used to treat distal femur fractures, there is still a role for dual plates for fractures with excessive comminution. Dual plating can be especially helpful for very short segment distal femoral articular blocks where an adequate number of screws cannot be placed through the plate or nail. Sanders and colleagues[52] report on a series of 9 patients who underwent dual plating for such fractures. They reported excellent union rates with significantly restricted knee motion. More recent studies have confirmed the benefits of dual plating for osteoporotic distal femur fractures.[53–55]

Another common place for the use of dual plating is the bicondylar tibial plateau fracture. Most of the patients with a tibial plateau fracture are older than 55 years, with a significant portion of them being bicondylar injuries.[56,57] Despite this information, there is a paucity of data on fracture fixation of the osteoporotic patient with a tibial plateau fracture. Su and colleagues[58] studied 38 patients with 39 plateau fractures in patients older than 55 years. They found while the majority of results were favorable, increasing age was associated with worse results. They did not study the use of dual plating in this situation. The studies looking at the use of dual plating for bicondylar injuries are not focused on the osteoporotic patient. Regardless, this technique has been shown to be associated with good outcomes.[59–61]

Nail-Plate Constructs

The use of the nail-plate combination for distal femur fractures and distal femoral nonunion is an effective way to achieve union. Attum and colleagues[62] reviewed 10 patients who underwent nail-plate constructs for femoral nonunion with reamer irrigator aspirator. Their results had a 100% union rate with only one deep infection. Spitler and colleagues[63] reported high union rates and low rates of secondary surgery in morbidly obese patients treated with a nail-plate construct. The benefit of a nail-plate construct is that it is a stiffer construct that can resist mechanical failure and can be helpful in

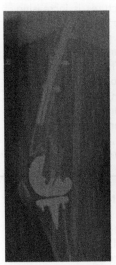
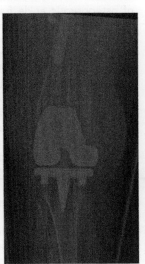
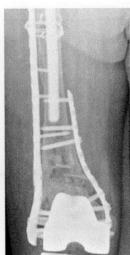
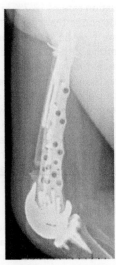

Fig. 2. A 63-year-old woman with injury and postoperative AP and lateral knee views demonstrating a dual plate construct for acute periprosthetic distal femur fracture.

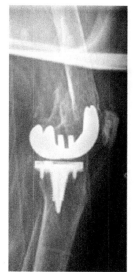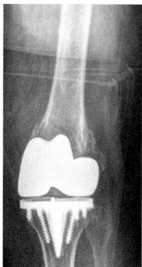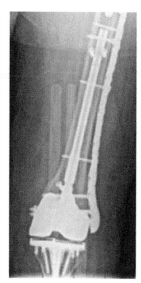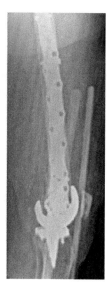

Fig. 3. A 91-year-old woman with injury and postoperative AP and lateral femur views demonstrating a nail-plate construct for acute periprosthetic distal femur fracture. Proximal blocking screws are placed to effectively narrow the intramedullary canal and reduce coronal toggle.

the setting of short articular segments with significant metaphyseal comminution (**Fig. 3**).

This same concept of nail-plate constructs has been used in both proximal and distal tibia fractures as well. Kubiak and colleagues[64] reviewed 24 patients who were treated with a nail-plate combination for a tibial plateau and ipsilateral tibial shaft fracture. They reported only one surgery for a delayed tibial shaft union and one below-knee amputation for failed soft tissue coverage of a grade IIIC open tibia fracture. Finally, Yoon and Liporace have outlined the use of the nail-plate construct in the distal tibia fracture.[65]

Blocking screws around the nail in the meta-diaphyseal or diaphyseal region can reduce the canal volume and prevent coronal toggle of the distal segment (see **Fig. 3**).[66] As previously stated, both distal femur and proximal tibias are common osteoporotic fractures; these types of interventions are important to remember when treating such fractures. Although these articles have shown promising results in the use of the nail-plate construct, no studies have specifically investigated the use of these implants in the osteoporotic patient.

Cement Augmentation

Cement augmentation is an important adjunct in osteoporotic fracture treatment, particularly with locked plate constructs. When angle-stable constructs fail, they commonly fail through cutout rather than pullout mechanism. Cement augmentation can significantly

strengthen screw purchase and potentially prevent cutout.[67]

Polymethyl methacrylate (PMMA) can be used to augment screw fixation in osteoporotic bone (**Fig. 4**). This strategy relies on the cement interdigitating with surrounding cancellous bone and creating a greater surface area. This environment results in stronger screw purchase after the cement polymerizes.[68] Early data on screw purchase within PMMA showed that axial screw pullout strength greatly increased in osteoporotic bone with PMMA augmentation.[69] In the trauma literature, PMMA supplementation has also shown increased load to failure. Goetzen and colleagues[70] evaluated PMMA augmentation in a cadaveric study of fixation of osteoporotic fracture with the LISS plate. They found that the nonaugmented group failed at approximately 9,417 load cycles compared with the PMMA augmented group that failed at approximately 14,792 load cycles ($P = .002$). Similar findings have been found in augmented fixation in the proximal femur and proximal humerus.[71]

PMMA augmentation has associated complications. The drying process of PMMA is an exothermic process and can lead to thermal necrosis of the surrounding bone and soft tissue. In vitro, this process can reach temperatures up to 113°C and in vivo temperatures have been demonstrated at between 40°C and 56°C.[72–74] PMMA is a permanent, nonbiological implant within the bone. In the case of revision surgery, the cement may need to be removed, which can be tedious and destructive to surrounding

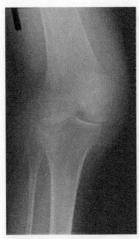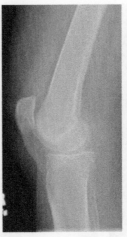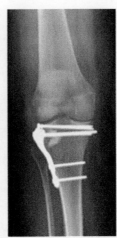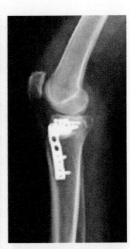

Fig. 4. A 83-year-old woman with injury and postoperative AP and lateral knee views demonstrating locking plate fixation augmented with PMMA in the bony defect.

tissue. Poorly placed cement could theoretically prevent bone healing at the site of a fracture because it does not promote or support bone growth.

Calcium sulfate and calcium phosphate cement are additional augments that can be used to increase screw purchase in patients with poor bone quality. These augments carry the advantage of supporting de novo bone healing and having nonexothermic curing processes. Both act as osteoconductive agents, and it has been shown when they are placed in a stable position adjacent to bone, osteoid is formed without interposed soft tissue.[67] Furthermore, these bone substitutes show better compressive strength than cancellous bone of good quality. One major advantage of calcium phosphate when compared with calcium sulfate is that as a result of the remodeling mechanism, calcium phosphate is not resorbed until new bone is being formed.[67] An osteoporotic bone model created by Stadelmann and colleagues[75] demonstrated maximum pullout strength of approximately 30 N. With the addition of calcium phosphate cement, the maximum pullout strength of the same cancellous screws could increase up to 1000 N depending on cement technique. Calcium sulfate cement augmentation used in lumbar vertebral bodies has approximately 167% increased pullout strength of pedicle screws compared with native bone.[76] Collinge and colleagues[77] evaluated locked plate fixation and standard plate fixation in osteoporotic bone with and without cement augmentation. Their model showed that cement augmentation with PMMA or tricalcium phosphate increased screw pullout strength by 3.6

times for standard plates and 3.3 times for locked plate. The strongest construct of all was the locked plate in osteoporotic model with cement augmentation, which was 5 times stronger at resisting pullout failure than the standard plate with no augmentation. As mentioned previously, when BMD falls below 0.4 g/cm^3, alterations in screw geometry and size are inconsequential. In this setting, cement augmentation could be critical to implant stability.[21]

NEW TECHNOLOGIES

With an aging population and increasing rate of fragility fractures, new technologies and creative ways to treat these injuries are gaining attention. Several techniques that show promise include hydroxyapatite-coated implants, polyaxial locking plates, far cortical locking, and improved screw design.

Hydroxyapatite-coated external fixator pins have shown promise in animal and clinical trials at increasing fixation in osteoporotic bone.[78] They function by increasing osteointegration and increasing strength at the bone-screw interface. Moroni and colleagues[79] also showed that 4.5 cortical screws coated with hydroxyapatite required an order of magnitude increase in extraction force for screw removal at 1 month after insertion. Recent in vivo data suggest that screws augmented with zoledronate-loaded nanohydroxyapatite particles demonstrate increased bone formation around screws.[80] These techniques need more investigation in the clinical setting.

Polyaxial locking plates were developed to aid in management of various complex fractures.

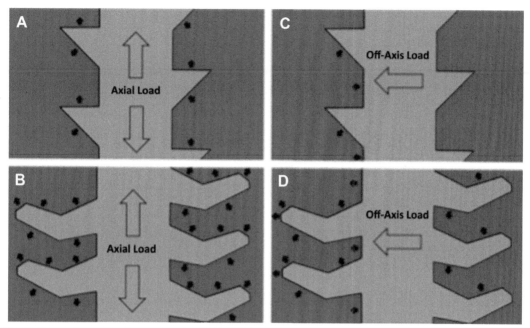

Fig. 5. Comparison of load vectors on the (B, D) SMV Bone–Screw-Fastener compared with the (A, C) conventional buttress thread resulting from axial load and off-axis load. (Courtesy of OsteoCentric Technologies, Austin, TX.)

They allow a conical trajectory of screws that still lock into the plate. The polyaxial locking plates enable increased flexibility in screw trajectory and screw fixation in multiple planes. In a biomechanical study of distal femur fractures, Wilkens and colleagues[81] found that polyaxial locking plates had a significantly higher load to failure than traditional locking plates. The polyaxial screws can be particularly helpful in treating osteoporotic periprosthetic fractures to allow for locking screw placement around any arthroplasty stems.

A new advance in screw design is promising for increasing fixation in osteoporotic bone. The Bone–Screw-Fastener (SMV Scientific) uses a unique thread design that is manufactured to resist multidirectional forces and bending moments (Fig. 5). The thread design resists both toggle and axial pullout better than standard screws. The screw design is also thought to have less possibility of stripping in patients with poor bone quality.[82] Finally, the bone cutting mechanism is designed to curl bone chips away from the cutting edge, which effectively reduces the amount of bone destruction during screw insertion. This screw design has been used clinically with success in fracture fixation, but randomized control trials and further biomechanical testing are needed to prove efficacy.

Modulating construct stiffness has become an important area of interest with the widespread

acceptance of locking plates. A potential disadvantage of locking plate fixation is making a construct with a stiffness profile that does not align with the mode of healing the surgeon is attempting to achieve. In most situations, this translates to creating a construct that is too stiff to achieve secondary bone healing, thus generating nonunion. Far cortical locking screws are

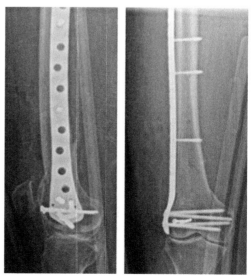

Fig. 6. A 76-year-old woman with postoperative AP and lateral femur views demonstrating far cortical locking screws.

a new technology that allows micromotion at the fracture site in the setting of a locking plate (Fig. 6). This technology shows a 54% increase in torsional strength, up to 21% increase in bending strength, and 84% of the compressive strength when compared with conventional locking plates.[83] In biomechanical studies, this technology was just as durable as standard locked plates. Most importantly, these constructs showed an increase rate of callus formation at the fracture site by approximately 36% overall callus volume.[84] Clinically, Linn and colleagues[85] demonstrated increase callus formation in distal femur fractures fixed with dynamic locking plates compared with standard locking plates. They used a technique of over drilling the near cortex to create a dynamic environment for fracture healing.

SUMMARY

The incidence of osteoporotic fracture is increasing with the aging US population. Because osteoporosis leads to a decrease in BMD with a decrease in both trabecular and cortical bone, osteoporotic fracture presents fixation challenges with standard plate and screw constructs. Locked plating has been developed to create a fixed-angle plate-screw construct that is more resistant to failure in osteoporotic bone. Endosteal replacement, additional plates, and cement augmentation have all been demonstrated to further supplement osteoporotic fracture fixation. Technologies on the horizon to treat osteoporotic fracture include SMV screws, hydroxyapatite-coated implants, and far cortical locking screws.

REFERENCES

1. America's Bone Health. The state of osteoporosis and low bone mass in our nation. Washington, DC: National Osteoporsis Foundation; 2002.
2. Wright NC, Looker AC, Saag KG, et al. The recent prevalence of osteoporosis and low bone mass in the United States based on bone mineral density at the femoral neck or lumbar spine. J Bone Miner Res 2014;29(11):2520–6.
3. Burge R, Dawson-hughes B, Solomon DH, et al. Incidence and economic burden of osteoporosis-related fractures in the United States, 2005-2025. J Bone Miner Res 2007;22(3):465–75.
4. Cenzer IS, Tang V, Boscardin WJ, et al. One-year mortality after hip fracture: development and validation of a prognostic index. J Am Geriatr Soc 2016;64(9):1893–8.
5. Braithwaite RS, Col NF, Wong JB. Estimating hip fracture morbidity, mortality and costs. J Am Geriatr Soc 2003;51(3):364–70.
6. Dell RM, Greene D, Anderson D, et al. Osteoporosis disease management: what every orthopaedic surgeon should know. J Bone Joint Surg Am 2009; 91(Suppl 6):79–86.
7. Cummings SR, Melton LJ. Epidemiology and outcomes of osteoporotic fractures. Lancet 2002; 359(9319):1761–7.
8. Browner BD, Jupiter JB, Krettek C, et al. Skeletal trauma, basic science, management, and reconstruction. Philadelphia: W.B. Saunders Company; 2003.
9. Parfitt AM. Trabecular bone architecture in the pathogenesis and prevention of fracture. Am J Med 1987;82(1B):68–72.
10. Fields AJ, Keaveny TM. Trabecular architecture and vertebral fragility in osteoporosis. Curr Osteoporos Rep 2012;10(2):132–40.
11. Snyder BD, Piazza S, Edwards WT, et al. Role of trabecular morphology in the etiology of age-related vertebral fractures. Calcif Tissue Int 1993; 53(Suppl 1):S14–22.
12. Schuit SC, Van der klift M, Weel AE, et al. Fracture incidence and association with bone mineral density in elderly men and women: the Rotterdam Study. Bone 2004;34(1):195–202.
13. Wainwright SA, Marshall LM, Ensrud KE, et al. Hip fracture in women without osteoporosis. J Clin Endocrinol Metab 2005;90(5):2787–93.
14. Riggs BL, Melton LJ iii, Robb RA, et al. Population-based study of age and sex differences in bone volumetric density, size, geometry, and structure at different skeletal sites. J Bone Miner Res 2004; 19(12):1945–54.
15. Yang L, Udall WJ, Mccloskey EV, et al. Distribution of bone density and cortical thickness in the proximal femur and their association with hip fracture in postmenopausal women: a quantitative computed tomography study. Osteoporos Int 2014;25(1):251–63.
16. Poole KE, Mayhew PM, Rose CM, et al. Changing structure of the femoral neck across the adult female lifespan. J Bone Miner Res 2010;25(3):482–91.
17. Rüedi TP, Buckley RE, Moran CG. AO principles of fracture management. Davos, Switzerland: AO Publishing; 2007.
18. Perren SM, Cordey J, Baumgart F, et al. Technical and biomechanical aspects of screws used for bone surgery. Int J Orthop Trauma;2:31–48.
19. Grant KD, Busse EC, Park DK, et al. Internal fixation of osteoporotic bone. J Am Acad Orthop Surg 2018;26(5):166–74.
20. Gardner MJ, Brophy RH, Campbell D, et al. The mechanical behavior of locking compression plates compared with dynamic compression plates in a

cadaver radius model. J Orthop Trauma 2005;19(9): 597–603.

21. Turner IG, Rice GN. Comparison of bone screw holding strength in healthy bovine and osteoporotic human cancellous bone. Clin Mater 1992;9: 105–7.

22. Borgeaud M, Cordey J, Leyvraz PE, et al. Mechanical analysis of the bone to plate interface of the LC-DCP and of the PC-FIX on human femora. Injury 2000;31(suppl 3):C29–36.

23. Kubiak EN, Fulkerson E, Strauss E, et al. The evolution of locked plates. J Bone Joint Surg Am 2006; 88(Suppl 4):189–200.

24. Cordey J, Borgeaud M, Perren SM. Force transfer between the plate and the bone: relative importance of the bending stiffness of the screws friction between plate and bone. Injury 2000;31(Suppl 3):C21–8.

25. Wehner T, Claes L, Simon U. Internal loads in the human tibia during gait. Clin Biomech (Bristol, Avon) 2009;24(3):299–302.

26. Egol KA, Kubiak EN, Fulkerson E, et al. Biomechanics of locked plates and screws. J Orthop Trauma 2004;18(8):488–93.

27. Ramotowski W, Granowski R. Zespol. An original method of stable osteosynthesis. Clin Orthop Relat Res 1991;(272):67–75.

28. Tepic S, Perren SM. The biomechanics of the PC-Fix internal fixator. Injury 1995;26(suppl 2):B5–10.

29. Anglen J, Kyle RF, Marsh JL, et al. Locking plates for extremity fractures. J Am Acad Orthop Surg 2009;17:465–72.

30. Rothberg DL, Lee MA. Internal fixation of osteoporotic fractures. Curr Osteoporos Rep 2015;13(1): 16–21.

31. Gautier E, Perren SM, Cordey J. Effect of plate position relative to bending direction on the rigidity of a plate osteosynthesis. A theoretical analysis. Injury 2000;31(suppl 3):C14–20.

32. Farouk O, Krettek C, Miclau T, et al. Effects of percutaneous and conventional plating techniques on the blood supply to the femur. Arch Orthop Trauma Surg 1998;117:438–41.

33. McLaurin TM. Proximal humerus fractures in the elderly are we operating on too many? Bull Hosp Jt Dis 2004;62:24–32.

34. Röderer G, Erhardt J, Graf M, et al. Clinical results for minimally invasive locked plating of proximal humerus fractures. J Orthop Trauma 2010;24(7): 400–6.

35. Kralinger F, Blauth M, Goldhahn J, et al. The influence of local bone density on the outcome of one hundred and fifty proximal humeral fractures treated with a locking plate. J Bone Joint Surg Am 2014;96(12):1026–32.

36. Olerud P, Ahrengart L, Ponzer S, et al. Internal fixation versus nonoperative treatment of displaced 3-part proximal humeral fractures in elderly patients: a randomized controlled trial. J Shoulder Elbow Surg 2011;20(5):747–55.

37. Südkamp N, Bayer J, Hepp P, et al. Open reduction and internal fixation of proximal humeral fractures with use of the locking proximal humerus plate. Results of a prospective, multicenter, observational study. J Bone Joint Surg Am 2009;91(6):1320–8.

38. Thanasas C, Kontakis G, Angoules A, et al. Treatment of proximal humerus fractures with locking plates: a systematic review. J Shoulder Elbow Surg 2009;18(6):837–44.

39. Little MTM, Berkes MB, Schottel PC, et al. The impact of preoperative coronal plane deformity on proximal humerus fixation with endosteal augmentation. J Orthop Trauma 2014;28(6):338–47.

40. Nellans KW, Kowalski E, Chung KC. The epidemiology of distal radius fractures. Hand Clin 2012; 28(2):113–25.

41. Karantana A, Downing ND, Forward DP, et al. Surgical treatment of distal radial fractures with a volar locking plate versus conventional percutaneous methods: a randomized controlled trial. J Bone Joint Surg Am 2013;95(19):1737–44.

42. Smith DW, Henry MH. Volar fixed-angle plating of the distal radius. J Am Acad Orthop Surg 2005; 13(1):28–36.

43. Wright TW, Horodyski M, Smith DW. Functional outcome of unstable distal radius fractures: ORIF with a volar fixed-angle tine plate versus external fixation. J Hand Surg Am 2005;30(2):289–99.

44. Jakubietz RG, Gruenert JG, Kloss DF, et al. A randomised clinical study comparing palmar and dorsal fixed-angle plates for the internal fixation of AO C-type fractures of the distal radius in the elderly. J Hand Surg Eur Vol 2008;33(5):600–4.

45. Ruckenstuhl P, Bernhardt GA, Sadoghi P, et al. Quality of life after volar locked plating: a 10-year follow-up study of patients with intra-articular distal radius fractures. BMC Musculoskelet Disord 2014; 15:250.

46. Lichtman DM, Bindra RR, Boyer MI, et al. American Academy of Orthopaedic Surgeons clinical practice guideline on: the treatment of distal radius fractures. J Bone Joint Surg Am 2011;93(8):775–8.

47. Haidukewych G, Sems SA, Huebner D, et al. Results of polyaxial locked-plate fixation of periarticular fractures of the knee. J Bone Joint Surg Am 2007; 89(3):614–20.

48. Kregor PJ, Stannard JA, Zlowodzki M, et al. Treatment of distal femur fractures using the less invasive stabilization system: surgical experience and early clinical results in 103 fractures. J Orthop Trauma 2004;18(8):509–20.

49. Ricci WM, Streubel PN, Morshed S, et al. Risk factors for failure of locked plate fixation of distal femur fractures: an analysis of 335 cases. J Orthop Trauma 2014;28(2):83–9.

50. Kannus P, Palvanen M, Niemi S, et al. Increasing number and incidence of low-trauma ankle fractures in elderly people: finnish statistics during 1970-2000 and projections for the future. Bone 2002;31:430–3.

51. Panchbhavi VK, Vallurupalli S, Morris R. Comparison of augmentation methods for internal fixation of osteoporotic ankle fractures. Foot Ankle Int 2009;30(7):696–703.

52. Sanders R, Swiontkowski M, Rosen H, et al. Double-plating of comminuted, unstable fractures of the distal part of the femur. J Bone Joint Surg Am 1991;73(3):341–6.

53. Steinberg EL, Elis J, Steinberg Y, et al. A double-plating approach to distal femur fracture: a clinical study. Injury 2017;48(10):2260–5.

54. Ziran BH, Rohde RH, Wharton AR. Lateral and anterior plating of intra-articular distal femoral fractures treated via an anterior approach. Int Orthop 2002; 26(6):370–3.

55. Holzman MA, Hanus BD, Munz JW, et al. Addition of a medial locking plate to an in situ lateral locking plate results in healing of distal femoral nonunions. Clin Orthop Relat Res 2016;474(6):1498–505.

56. Rasmussen PS. Tibial condylar fractures. Impairment of knee joint stability as an indication for surgical treatment. J Bone Joint Surg Am 1973;55(7):1331–50.

57. Rozell JC, Vemulapalli KC, Gary JL, et al. Tibial plateau fractures in elderly patients. Geriatr Orthop Surg Rehabil 2016;7(3):126–34.

58. Su EP, Westrich GH, Rana AJ, et al. Operative treatment of tibial plateau fractures in patients older than 55 years. Clin Orthop Relat Res 2004;421: 240–8.

59. Zhang P, Lian K, Luo D, et al. A combined approach for the treatment of lateral and posterolateral tibial plateau fractures. Injury 2016;47(10):2326–30.

60. Ozkaya U, Parmaksizoglu AS. Dual locked plating of unstable bicondylar tibial plateau fractures. Injury 2015;46(Suppl 2):S9–13.

61. Barei DP, Nork SE, Mills WJ, et al. Functional outcomes of severe bicondylar tibial plateau fractures treated with dual incisions and medial and lateral plates. J Bone Joint Surg Am 2006;88(8):1713–21.

62. Attum B, Douleh D, Whiting PS, et al. Outcomes of distal femur nonunions treated with a combined nail/plate construct and autogenous bone grafting. J Orthop Trauma 2017;31(9):e301–4.

63. Spitler CA, Bergin PF, Russell GV, et al. Endosteal substitution with an intramedullary rod in fractures of the femur. J Orthop Trauma 2018;32(Suppl 1):S25–9.

64. Kubiak EN, Camuso MR, Barei DP, et al. Operative treatment of ipsilateral noncontiguous unicondylar tibial plateau and shaft fractures: combining plates and nails. J Orthop Trauma 2008;22(8):560–5.

65. Yoon RS, Liporace FA. Intramedullary nail and plate combination fixation for complex distal tibia fractures: when and how? J Orthop Trauma 2016; 30(Suppl 4):S17–21.

66. Auston D, Donohue D, Stoops K, et al. Long segment blocking screws increase the stability of retrograde nail fixation in geriatric supracondylar femur fractures: eliminating the "bell-clapper effect". J Orthop Trauma 2018;32(11):559–64.

67. Larsson S, Stadelmann VA, Arnoldi J, et al. Injectable calcium phosphate cement for augmentation around cancellous bone screws. In vivo biomechanical studies. J Biomech 2012;45(7):1156–60.

68. Jaeblon T. Polymethylmethacrylate: properties and contemporary uses in orthopaedics. J Am Acad Orthop Surg 2010;18(5):297–305.

69. Cameron HU, Jacob R, Macnab I, et al. Use of polymethylmethacrylate to enhance screw fixation in bone. J Bone Joint Surg Am 1975;57(5):655–6.

70. Goetzen M, Nicolino T, Hofmann-fliri L, et al. Metaphyseal screw augmentation of the LISS-PLT plate with polymethylmethacrylate improves angular stability in osteoporotic proximal third tibial fractures: a biomechanical study in human cadaveric tibiae. J Orthop Trauma 2014;28(5):294–9.

71. Sermon A, Hofmann-fliri L, Richards RG, et al. Cement augmentation of hip implants in osteoporotic bone: how much cement is needed and where should it go? J Orthop Res 2014;32(3):362–8.

72. Kuehn KD, Ege W, Gopp U. Acrylic bone cements: composition and properties. Orthop Clin North Am 2005;36:17–28.

73. Belkoff SM, Molloy S. Temperature measurement during polymerization of polymethylmethacrylate cement used for vertebroplasty. Spine (Phila Pa 1976) 2003;28:1555–9.

74. Webb JC, Spencer RF. The role of polymethylmethacrylate bone cement in modern orthopaedic surgery. J Bone Joint Surg Br 2007;89:851–7.

75. Stadelmann VA, Bretton E, Terrier A, et al. Calcium phosphate cement augmentation of cancellous bone screws can compensate for the absence of cortical fixation. J Biomech 2010;43(15):2869–74.

76. Rohmiller MT, Schwalm D, Glattes RC, et al. Evaluation of calcium sulfate paste for augmentation of lumbar pedicle screw pullout strength. Spine J 2002;2:255–60.

77. Collinge C, Merk B, Lautenschlager EP. Mechanical evaluation of fracture fixation augmented with tricalcium phosphate bone cement in a porous osteoporotic cancellous bone model. J Orthop Trauma 2007;21(2):124–8.

78. Moroni A, Vannini F, Mosca M, et al. State of the art review: techniques to avoid pin loosening and infection in external fixation. J Orthop Trauma 2002;16(3):189–95.

79. Moroni A, Aspenberg P, Toksvig-Larsen S, et al. Enhanced fixation with hydroxyapatite coated pins. Clin Orthop 1998;346:171–7.

80. Kettenberger U, Luginbuehl V, Procter P, et al. In vitro and in vivo investigation of bisphosphonate-loaded

hydroxyapatite particles for peri-implant bone augmentation. J Tissue Eng Regen Med 2017;11(7): 1974–85.

81. Wilkens KJ, Curtiss S, Lee MA. Polyaxial locking plate fixation in distal femur fractures: a biomechanical comparison. J Orthop Trauma 2008;22(9): 624–8.

82. Stahel PF, Alfonso NA, Henderson C, et al. Introducing the "Bone-Screw-Fastener" for improved screw fixation in orthopedic surgery: a revolutionary paradigm shift? Patient Saf Surg 2017;11:6.

83. Bottlang M, Doornink J, Lujan TJ, et al. Effects of construct stiffness on healing of fractures stabilized with locking plates. J Bone Joint Surg Am 2010; 92(Suppl 2):12–22.

84. Lujan TJ, Henderson CE, Madey SM, et al. Locked plating of distal femur fractures leads to inconsistent and asymmetric callus formation. J Orthop Trauma 2010;24:156–62.

85. Linn MS, Mcandrew CM, Prusaczyk B, et al. Dynamic locked plating of distal femur fractures. J Orthop Trauma 2015;29(10):447–50.

Vitamin D and Metabolic Supplementation in Orthopedic Trauma

Samantha Nino, MD[a], Sandeep P. Soin, MD[a],
Frank R. Avilucea, MD[b],*

KEYWORDS

- Vitamin D • Hypovitaminosis D • Fracture healing • Fracture nonunion
- Vitamin D supplementation • Metabolic • Endocrine

KEY POINTS

- This article provides a general background on the metabolic role of vitamin D in musculoskeletal health.
- The authors discuss the widespread prevalence of hypovitaminosis D, risk factors, and biologic consequences.
- The authors review pertinent literature regarding vitamin D supplementation, it's controversial role in fracture prevention and healing, and available guidelines for supplementation.
- The authors briefly review other metabolic and endocrine considerations in the trauma patient including calcium intake, vitamin K, and hormone analogue therapy.

INTRODUCTION

Nutritional supplementation has gained increasing attention in the general public and in health care. Calcium and vitamin D have received notable attention, particularly as pertains to fracture healing, fracture prevention, and the role in treatment of osseous nonunions. The role of other supplements or medications in musculoskeletal health has also been investigated. These include vitamin K and anabolic hormone analogues.

This article serves as an overview for the role of metabolic supplementation and effects of specific medications on musculoskeletal health in the orthopedic trauma patient. The focus is on vitamin D and calcium, and vitamin K, medications, and endocrine considerations.

VITAMIN D

Background

Vitamin D is a subclass of fat-soluble steroids and is essential to calcium, phosphate, and parathyroid hormone (PTH) homeostasis in the human body. Although the term vitamin D is used broadly, it is typically used to describe the forms of vitamin D that are available through diet: cholecalciferol (vitamin D_3) and ergocalciferol (vitamin D_2). Unlike conventional vitamins, calciferol is not exclusively acquired through diet. This fat-soluble steroid is unique in that it can also be synthesized by the skin. Cutaneous production results from the conversion of 7-dehydrocholesterol to cholecalciferol via ultraviolet B (UVB) radiation, which is available from ambient sun exposure (**Fig. 1**).

Cholecalciferol is biologically inert, requiring hydroxylation by the liver to produce 25-hydroxycholecalciferol, referred to as calcifediol or calcidiol. This is the form of vitamin D that is measured clinically to characterize vitamin D sufficiency; however, this form of the vitamin requires renal hydroxylation to yield 1,25-hydroxycholecalciferol, called calcitriol (see **Fig. 1**). Calcitriol is the biologically active hormonal

[a] Department of Orthopaedics, Orlando Health, Orlando Health Orthopaedic Institute, 1222 South Orange Avenue, MP 43, Orlando, FL 32806, USA; [b] Level One Orthopedics, Orlando Health, Orlando Health Orthopaedic Institute, 1222 South Orange Avenue, MP 43, Orlando, FL 32806, USA
* Corresponding author.
E-mail address: favilucea@gmail.com

Orthop Clin N Am 50 (2019) 171–179
https://doi.org/10.1016/j.ocl.2018.12.001
0030-5898/19/© 2018 Elsevier Inc. All rights reserved.

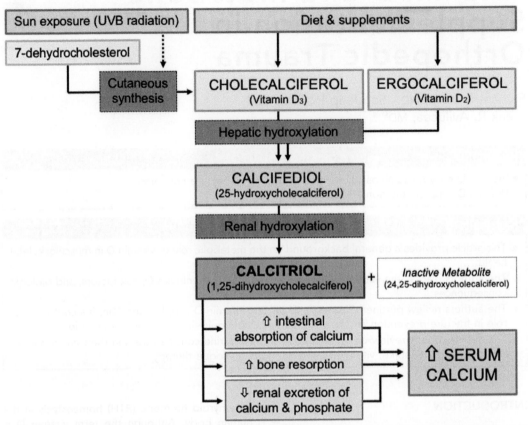

Fig. 1. Cholecalciferol and ergocalciferol are obtained from dietary sources and additional cholecalciferol is synthesized in the skin converted from 7-dehydrocholesterol and activated by UVB radiation. Cholecalciferol undergoes hydroxylation in the liver to form calcifediol, which undergoes hydroxylation in the kidneys to form the active form of vitamin D, calcitriol, and an inactive metabolite. Increased calcitriol levels lead to the activation of multiple pathways, which all function to ultimately increase serum calcium concentration in the body.

form of vitamin D and is among a small subclass of anabolic steroids known as secosteroids. Secosteroids have a broken-ring molecular structure (**Fig. 2**) and therefore calcitriol shares a form and mechanism of action similar to other hormones. Renal production of calcitriol is closely regulated by calcium, and thus PTH.

Although sun exposure may yield sufficient vitamin D levels, this method of managing vitamin D insufficiency is not favorable because season and geographic latitude may preclude appropriate UVB exposure. Additionally, because of the potential carcinogenic effects of UVB, increased exposure to this source is not pursued. As such, dietary supplementation is the preferred method for managing low vitamin D levels.

Prevalence of Vitamin D Deficiency/ Insufficiency

Experts contend that serum levels of calcifediol (25-hydroxycholecalciferol) less than 32 ng/mL

is a biologically significant threshold for vitamin D insufficiency because levels lower than this threshold result in decreased intestinal absorption of calcium and therefore increased synthesis and secretion of PTH.[1] PTH secretion leads to increased renal activation of calcifediol, renal reabsorption of calcium, and mobilization of bone calcium, physiologic changes striving to maintain normocalcemia.[2] If levels further fall lower than 20 ng/mL then there is no longer enough substrate to form biologically active calcitriol (1,25-dihydroxycholecalciferol), thus 20 ng/mL is considered the threshold for deficiency.[1] Without calcitriol the intestinal absorption of calcium has been shown to be reduced by up to 50%, resulting in maximal PTH secretion as the body attempts to maintain necessary ratios of calcium and phosphate within the collagen matrix needed for adequate bone mineralization.[1,2] Prolonged vitamin D deficiency results in acquired secondary hyperparathyroidism, which can progress to the

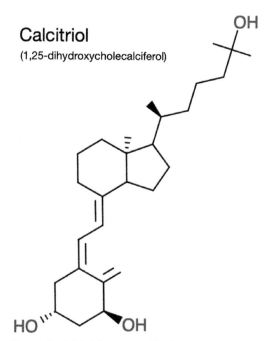

Calcitriol

(1,25-dihydroxycholecalciferol)

Fig. 2. Calcitriol (1,25-dihydroxycholecalciferol) demonstrating the broken ring molecular structure typical of secosteroids.

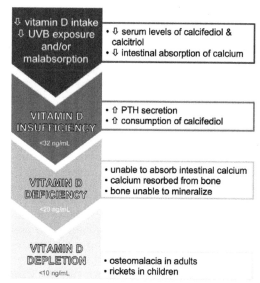

Fig. 3. When impaired vitamin D intake results in calcifediol levels less than 32 ng/mL, PTH is secreted, and the consumption of calcifediol increases as it is converted to active calcitriol; this results in further reduction in calcifediol concentration less than 20 ng/mL. Lower than this level is considered deficiency, which means intestinal absorption of calcium is severely impaired, more calcium is resorbed from bone stores, and bone is thus unable to be mineralized. When calcifediol levels fall less than 10 ng/mL it is considered depletion and if it is persistent can manifest clinically as osteomalacia in adults and rickets in children.

development of osteomalacia in adults and rickets in children (**Fig. 3**).

Vitamin D deficiency is a global concern and awareness of its prevalence has grown in recent years. The US National Health and Nutrition Examination Survey data showed nearly 70% of participants with serum calcifediol levels lower than 30 ng/mL.[3] Researchers estimate that 1 billion people worldwide are either vitamin D insufficient or deficient, including more than half of postmenopausal women with osteoporosis and even up to 36% of healthy 18- to 29-year-old adults.[4,5] Limited sun exposure for cutaneous synthesis, low dietary intake of vitamin D, and an assortment of risk factors have contributed to this rampant global vitamin deficiency.

Risk factors for hypovitaminosis D (serum concentration of 25-hydroxycholecalciferol <32 ng/mL) have been found to include: obesity; nutritional malabsorption; hepatic and renal disease; increasing latitudes; use of sunscreen; increasing age; and a variety of medications including cholesterol-lowering drugs, glucocorticoids, and antiepileptics (**Box 1**).[3] The half-life of vitamin D is approximately 30 days so serum levels tend to drop rapidly across the autumn and winter months, when sun exposure and thus cutaneous vitamin D synthesis decrease substantially.[6] Furthermore, individuals often overestimate their exposure to sunlight and one study found that even in a group of athletes

with daily sun exposure, 56% had calcifediol levels considered deficient (<32 ng/mL).[7]

In addition to the systemic effects of vitamin D, increasing evidence posits the potential benefits of the vitamin to skeletal health and function. For all of these reasons, vitamin D is of particular interest to orthopedic trauma surgeons and their patients.

Screening Programs

Because there is still no consensus regarding vitamin D supplementation, it should not be

| Box 1 |
Risk factors for hypovitaminosis D
Obesity
Intestinal malabsorption
Poor nutritional intake
Hepatic or renal disease
Old age
Use of sunscreen
Living at higher latitudes

surprising to find that there are no strong guidelines for screening for hypovitaminosis D. The Endocrine Society reports that optimal calcifediol levels may be gender- and age-dependent, but supplementation goals and guidelines should revolve around minimizing PTH secretion.[8] At this time, the most widely accepted laboratory assay is the measurement of calcifediol, or 25-hydroxycholecalciferol, levels. The threshold for vitamin D insufficiency is broadly accepted as calcifediol serum concentrations lower than 32 ng/mL, whereas deficiency is defined by concentrations lower than 20 ng/mL. As research findings continue to emerge, physicians of all disciplines await reliable markers to assess vitamin D adequacy and concise treatment and screening guidelines. A practical approach for the orthopedic surgeon is to screen patients for hypovitaminosis D in the setting of fragility fracture or delayed fracture healing or nonunion.[9]

Role in Musculoskeletal Health

There have been several recent studies demonstrating a relationship between vitamin D deficiency and athletic performance. A specific vitamin D receptor (VDR) discovered in skeletal muscle has led researchers to explore the potential of vitamin D supplementation to affect muscle function, strength, and recovery. Vitamin D promotes muscle cell proliferation and differentiation via VDR. It has also been shown to enhance movement of myosin over actin within the sarcomere, which can result in greater contractile force of the muscle unit.[10] Moreover, animal studies demonstrate that mice without functional VDRs have smaller and more variable muscle fiber size, lower body weight, size, and coordination compared with wild-type.[11]

Multiple randomized controlled trials have found statistically significant improvements in muscle strength with increased daily vitamin D intake.[10] Notably, a randomized placebo-controlled trial demonstrated a positive effect of supplementation on sprint times and vertical jump heights. The supplemented group received 5000 IU per day over an 8-week period, and at the end of the trial recorded substantially increased vertical heights, whereas no change was observed in the placebo group. A total of 70% of the studied population was baseline-deficient, with calcifediol levels lower than 20 ng/mL at the start of the trial.[12]

As the link between vitamin D intake and neuromuscular coordination is further defined, some authors currently extrapolate that vitamin D may have an important role in reducing the incidence of falls in high-risk geriatric populations.[3]

Role in Fracture Prevention

Vitamin D has a central role in bone metabolism that is well established. It has recently been suggested to have a significant role in fracture risk, fracture healing, incidence of falls, and neuromuscular control.[3] A 2005 meta-analysis of randomized controlled trials compared oral supplementation of vitamin D, with and without calcium, with placebo in older adults and determined that daily vitamin D supplementation reduced the relative risk of hip fractures by 26%.[13] A 2009 Cochrane review then concluded that vitamin D supplementation, although not effective in preventing fractures alone, but coupled with calcium did reduce the risk of hip fractures in elderly patients receiving institutional care.[14] Another meta-analysis of patients older than 50 years old supplemented with at least 800 IU of vitamin D and 1200 mg of calcium showed a pooled reduction in all fractures of 12%.[15] However, a recent, large meta-analysis, published in the endocrinology literature, compiled data from 81 variable studies and concluded that vitamin D supplementation does not prevent fractures or have any significant effect on bone mineral density.[16] This disconnect in the body of literature requires additional physician scrutiny when creating clinical protocols. Overall, especially given the amount of conflicted meta-analyses, it is too soon for the medical community to make a concrete recommendation regarding the benefits of vitamin D supplementation, which are discussed more in depth later in this article.

Considering the prevalence of hypovitaminosis D in nonfragility fracture patients was found to be 77.5%, it is important that orthopedic traumatologists remain up-to-date with interest in continued vitamin D research.[17] Despite the discrepancies in the literature regarding the effect of vitamin D on bone mineral density there is a compelling basic science connection between bone architecture and vitamin D. An analysis of iliac crest biopsies demonstrated an association between vitamin D deficiency and a decrease in number of viable osteocytes in cortical and cancellous bone.[18] However, there is a still a paucity of well-powered clinical studies to demonstrate a clinically meaningful effect.

Role in Fracture Healing

Endocrinology studies initially demonstrated the importance of cholecalciferol in early fracture healing and callous formation.[19] In osteoporotic rat models with fractured femurs, daily calcitriol administration resulted in significantly increased bone biomechanical strength.[20] In adult orthopedic trauma patients it has been shown that the incidence of delayed union is higher in those who are vitamin D deficient at the time of injury and persistently deficient through the post-fracture healing period.[21] Unfortunately, it is difficult to make conclusions regarding the effect of vitamin D supplementation in the trauma population. Because of high fracture union rates independent of vitamin D status, studies would require extremely large numbers to show the effect of vitamin D on fracture union. Furthermore, it has been postulated that the defined thresholds for vitamin D insufficiency and deficiency may not actually be clinically relevant to fracture healing, especially with fractures at low risk for nonunion.[22]

Implications in Nonunion

Many studies, and subsequent metanalyses, continue to demonstrate that there is insufficient evidence to support that hypovitaminosis D has implications in fracture nonunion.

A study that linked vitamin D deficiency to risk of fracture nonunion found that 68% of patients with fracture nonunions were calcifediol deficient.[9] However, that prevalence is similar to the observed rate of hypovitaminosis D in the general orthopedic trauma population.[23,24]

It is unlikely that vitamin D deficiency is the root cause of nonunion. Rather, the rampant prevalence of hypovitaminosis D is probably a contributing factor putting patients at higher risk of fracture nonunion.

Guidelines for Supplementation

There has been debate among experts regarding vitamin D supplementation guidelines. The Institute of Medicine recommends 400 IU daily, whereas the Endocrine Society argues for 2000 IU supplementation daily to achieve serum calcifediol levels associated with optimal calcium and PTH homeostasis.[8] A 2018 multicenter study of 259 adult orthopedic trauma patients compared these competing recommendations. They found that daily supplementation with 2000 IU was more effective at maintaining calcifediol levels higher than 30 ng/mL, versus 400 IU daily.[25] The study also demonstrated that for every 100-IU increase in supplementation there is an associated 8% decrease in risk of vitamin D deficiency.[25] Other recent orthopedic meta-analyses have similarly suggested that daily doses higher than 1000 IU may be most efficacious.[17]

A recent study on the efficacy of supplementation was conducted with an orthopedic trauma population. Vitamin D–deficient patients with an array of traumatic fractures were instructed to take twice daily vitamin D_3 with oral calcium supplements, which were provided free of cost. All of the patients that were compliant with supplementation were able to correct their initial vitamin D deficiency to normal levels after a mean of 7 weeks.[26]

Although most of this article focuses on supplementation it is worth mentioning the other sources of vitamin D that are readily available to patients: food and sun exposure. The US Dietary Guidelines for Americans currently recommends 600 IU daily for the average American to maintain already adequate serum levels of vitamin D.[27] Most commonly recommended food sources (**Box 2**) include fatty fish, fortified dairy products, and eggs. Salmon and trout have some of the highest concentrations of vitamin D_3 available from a food source.[6] Fortified dairy products, such as milk and cheese, are readily available and affordable sources for most patients. Cutaneous synthesis is a nondietary source of cholecalciferol, but it tends to be inadequate as the principal source of vitamin D for most people. Prolonged sun exposure is necessary to synthesize enough vitamin D to avoid hypovitaminosis D. American public health authorities have long fought for the avoidance of prolonged sun exposure because of known association of UV radiation and the development of melanoma.[28] Encouraging regular sun exposure to treat hypovitaminosis D is likely insufficient and one would need to balance any benefit with the risk associated with UV radiation exposure.

According to the US Preventative Services Task Force, current evidence is still insufficient to adequately balance the benefits and harms of vitamin D supplementation for the primary prevention of fractures in healthy adults.[29] Conflicting conclusions regarding the benefits of

Box 2 Common dietary sources of vitamin D
Tuna
Salmon
Trout
Fortified dairy
Cheese
Egg yolk

vitamin D supplements, or lack thereof, requires physicians to critically analyze the risk benefit margin for each patient. Over-the-counter vitamin D supplements are low cost to the patient and complications related to toxicity are rare. The few reports of severe vitamin intoxication were attributable to manufacturer errors. Two patients were documented to have consumed nearly 1,000,000 IU daily for 1 month and found to have calcifediol concentrations greater than 1000 ng/mL.[10] Symptoms of vitamin D toxicity were secondary to hypercalcemia and included anorexia, polydipsia, polyuria, nausea, and in the most severe cases renal impairment.[10,17] It has been demonstrated that serums levels greater than 300 ng/mL are associated with toxicity, so the overall recommendation is that 100 ng/mL should be considered a safe upper limit of the normal range, which would retain a wide safety margin for toxicity.[30] The potential benefits of vitamin D adequacy in children and adults seem to outweigh the potential risks of deficiency. Orthopedic studies and meta-analyses have suggested that daily doses greater than 1000 IU may be most efficacious in treating hypovitaminosis D with a low risk of toxicity.[17,25]

OTHER METABOLIC CONSIDERATIONS
Calcium

Calcium metabolism is closely related to vitamin D because the two work synergistically. The skeleton acts as an important reservoir for blood calcium levels, which needs to remain tightly controlled. This is achieved through interaction of different hormones, including PTH, calcitonin, and vitamin D. Healthy bones continually turn over calcium and are constantly remodeling. To maintain a healthy bone structure, patients need a dietary source of calcium. The recommended daily allowance of dietary calcium from all sources is 1000 mg for men aged 19 to 70 years old and women aged 19 to 50 years old, and it increases to 1200 mg for women older than 50 years. The daily upper limit is 2500 mg up to age 50, then decreases to 2000 mg. These values represent calcium from all sources including dairy, meats, vegetables, and supplementation.[31]

An important element in maintaining adequate calcium serum concentrations is gastrointestinal absorption of calcium, which is limited to roughly 500 mg to 600 mg at a time. Therefore, patients requiring calcium supplementation are often advised to take a supplement twice daily. Absorption is also affected by cofactors, such as vitamin D, which is often added to dairy products and to many over-the-counter calcium supplements. The type of calcium compound is another aspect affecting calcium supplementation. The two most common formulations of calcium supplements are calcium carbonate (40% elemental calcium) and calcium citrate (21% elemental calcium). Although calcium carbonate contains more elemental calcium and is generally cheaper, it is not as well tolerated as calcium citrate. Absorption profiles are better with calcium citrate and supplementation has been shown to be associated with decreased markers of bone resorption, as compared with calcium carbonate supplementation.[32,33]

Careful attention is required in ensuring an appropriate level of calcium is consumed. In patients with a predilection of hypercalcemia or excess blood calcium, increased supplementation can lead to higher blood levels and subsequent arrhythmias or other untoward effects. Additionally, excess calcium supplementation results in increased urinary calcium and may result in increased risk for calcium oxalate nephrolithiasis.[34]

Vitamin K

Vitamin K is recognized as an important cofactor in the clotting cascade; however, it has received some attention recently for its role in musculoskeletal health. Vitamin K is a liposoluble vitamin discovered in 1929 for its central effect in the liver and on clot formation. Common sources of vitamin K include green, leafy vegetables and some fruits. Uniquely, it is also produced endogenously by bacteria within the bowel.

Vitamin K plays a role in maintaining bone strength by acting as a cofactor for gamma carboxylase, which subsequently activates multiple vitamin K–dependent proteins in bone, including osteocalcin, an important protein involved in osteoblast and osteoclast homeostasis. Others have postulated that vitamin K plays a direct role in regulating osteoclastogenesis and osteoblastogenesis through the NF-KappaB (NFKB) pathway.[35,36]

Despite these roles vitamin K has in bone turnover and regulation at a molecular level there is poor evidence to support intake and supplementation affecting molecular markers of bone turnover in patient populations. However, there have been studies that show patients with low vitamin K plasma level trended toward lower femoral neck bone mineral density (BMD). Interestingly, vitamin K antagonist, such as warfarin, may increase fracture risk. In a study of patients on warfarin for atrial fibrillation there was an increased serum RANKL level and in a separate study there was an association between males on warfarin and osteoporotic fractures.[37,38]

There is no consensus regarding vitamin K supplementation in patients with low serum vitamin K level or an evidence for limiting vitamin K antagonists in patients with osteoporosis or acute fracture. The evidence is currently lacking to make any recommendations to change clinical practice with regards to vitamin K. The basic science literature does support further investigation into the role of vitamin K in bone health.

ENDOCRINE CONSIDERATIONS

Fracture nonunion is a costly complication and when it occurs without a clear cause, it is reasonable to be suspicious that the patient may have a metabolic or endocrine abnormality. In a study of 638 nonunions, 37 of those were referred to an endocrinologist for evaluation because they met the following criteria:

1. Nonunion despite adequate reduction and stabilization of the fracture,
2. Multiple low-energy fractures with at least one progressing to nonunion, and/or
3. Nondisplaced pubic rami or sacral ala nonunion.

Of the 37 patients meeting one of those criteria, 83.8% were diagnosed with a metabolic or endocrine abnormality, most common of which was vitamin D deficiency.[9] Other derangements included calcium deficiency, hypogonadism, thyroid dysfunction, and parathyroid dysfunction. To assist in diagnosis, the following laboratory assays should be considered when evaluating for endocrine and metabolic derangements: 25-hydroxycholecalciferol, ionized calcium, PTH, alkaline phosphatase, phosphorus, thyroid-stimulating hormone, and/or free testosterone. Ultimately, orthopedic traumatologists should be prepared to refer patients meeting the previously mentioned criteria to an endocrinologist for further evaluation.

Teriparatide
Hormone analogues, such as teriparatide, have been used for the treatment of osteoporosis. Teriparatide and abaloparatide are considered anabolic therapies because they promote new bone formation via activation of PTH receptors. They are both administered via daily subcutaneous injection and have been shown to decrease the incidence of vertebral and nonvertebral fractures in postmenopausal osteoporotic women.[39]

In rat models, abaloparatide therapy generated a dose-dependent increase in the structural strength of vertebral bodies, femoral necks, and femoral shafts.[40] Recent clinical studies have demonstrated similar results in postmenopausal osteoporotic patients who received anabolic therapy for 18 months.[41] There have been case series and reports of "off-label" use of teriparatide in fracture nonunion and delayed union.[42,43] Although these hormone analogues have not been well studied in regard to orthopedic trauma, it seems there is a wealth of potential that can be extrapolated for anabolic therapy to play a role in fracture healing.

SUMMARY

A burgeoning wealth of scientific literature recognizes the potential musculoskeletal benefits of vitamin D supplementation, and the consequences of insufficiency and deficiency. It is therefore recommended that orthopedic surgeons assume a role in the diagnosis and treatment of patients with potential vitamin D deficiency. Disappointingly, current evidence is still too insufficient to prescribe optimal serum concentrations of calcifediol in orthopedic trauma patients, but it is hoped that future research will focus on identifying reliable markers to assess vitamin D adequacy and subsequently guide patient care with concise evidence-based treatment guidelines. Nonetheless, active assessment and management of hypovitaminosis D among the orthopedic patient population is low risk and low cost with significant potential to ultimately improve patient care. Adequate calcium intake is essential to maintaining healthy bone turnover and there are well-established guidelines on appropriate calcium intake, which can be of either a dietary or supplemental source. The current literature on the effects of vitamin K on bone health is limited but there may be some clinical role as more is learned. Aside from screening for endocrine abnormalities there is currently no role for endocrine supplementation in the otherwise healthy trauma patient. Currently the use of teriparatide is not approved for nonunion or delayed union; however, case reports have shown positive results in recalcitrant cases of nonunion.

REFERENCES

1. Hollis BW. Circulating 25-hydroxyvitamin D levels indicative of vitamin D sufficiency: implications for establishing a new effective dietary intake recommendation for vitamin D. J Nutr 2005;135(2): 317–22.

2. DeLuca HF. Overview of general physiologic features and functions of vitamin D. Am J Clin Nutr 2004;80(6 Suppl):1689S–96S.

3. Patton CM, Powell AP, Patel AA. Vitamin D in orthopaedics. J Am Acad Orthop Surg 2012;20(3): 123–9.

4. Tangpricha V, Pearce EN, Chen TC, et al. Vitamin D insufficiency among free-living healthy young adults. Am J Med 2002;112(8):659–62.

5. Holick MF. Vitamin D deficiency. N Engl J Med 2007;357(3):266–81.

6. Chen TC, Chimeh F, Lu Z, et al. Factors that influence the cutaneous synthesis and dietary sources of vitamin D. Arch Biochem Biophys 2007;460(2): 213–7.

7. Farrokhyar F, Tabasinejad R, Dao D, et al. Prevalence of vitamin D inadequacy in athletes: a systematic-review and meta-analysis. Sports Med 2015;45(3):365–78.

8. Holick MF, Binkley NC, Bischoff-Ferrari HA, et al. Guidelines for preventing and treating vitamin D deficiency and insufficiency revisited. J Clin Endocrinol Metab 2012;97(4):1153–8.

9. Brinker MR, O'Connor DP, Monla YT, et al. Metabolic and endocrine abnormalities in patients with nonunions. J Orthop Trauma 2007;21(8):557–70.

10. Abrams GD, Feldman D, Safran MR. Effects of vitamin D on skeletal muscle and athletic performance. J Am Acad Orthop Surg 2018;26(8): 278–85.

11. Endo I, Inoue D, Mitsui T, et al. Deletion of vitamin D receptor gene in mice results in abnormal skeletal muscle development with deregulated expression of myoregulatory transcription factors. Endocrinology 2003;144(12):5138–44.

12. Close GL, Russell J, Cobley JN, et al. Assessment of vitamin D concentration in non-supplemented professional athletes and healthy adults during the winter months in the UK: implications for skeletal muscle function. J Sports Sci 2013;31(4):344–53.

13. Bischoff-Ferrari HA, Willett WC, Wong JB, et al. Fracture prevention with vitamin D supplementation: a meta-analysis of randomized controlled trials. JAMA 2005;293(18):2257–64.

14. Avenell A, Gillespie WJ, Gillespie LD, et al. Vitamin D and vitamin D analogues for preventing fractures associated with involutional and post-menopausal osteoporosis. Cochrane Database Syst Rev 2009;(2):CD000227.

15. Tang BM, Eslick GD, Nowson C, et al. Use of calcium or calcium in combination with vitamin D supplementation to prevent fractures and bone loss in people aged 50 years and older: a meta-analysis. Lancet 2007;370(9588):657–66.

16. Bolland MJ, Grey A, Avenell A. Effects of vitamin D supplementation on musculoskeletal health: a systematic review, meta-analysis, and trial sequential analysis. Lancet Diabetes Endocrinol 2018;6(11): 847–58.

17. Sprague S, Petrisor B, Scott T, et al. What is the role of vitamin d supplementation in acute fracture patients? A systematic review and meta-analysis of the prevalence of hypovitaminosis D and supplementation efficacy. J Orthop Trauma 2016;30(2):53–63.

18. Rolvien T, Krause M, Jeschke A, et al. Vitamin D regulates osteocyte survival and perilacunar remodeling in human and murine bone. Bone 2017;103:78–87.

19. Lidor C, Dekel S, Edelstein S. The metabolism of vitamin D3 during fracture healing in chicks. Endocrinology 1987;120(1):389–93.

20. Fu L, Tang T, Miao Y, et al. Effect of 1,25-dihydroxy vitamin D3 on fracture healing and bone remodeling in ovariectomized rat femora. Bone 2009;44(5): 893–8.

21. Gorter EA, Krijnen P, Schipper IB. Vitamin D status and adult fracture healing. J Clin Orthop Trauma 2017;8(1):34–7.

22. Haines N, Kempton LB, Seymour RB, et al. The effect of a single early high-dose vitamin D supplement on fracture union in patients with hypovitaminosis D: a prospective randomised trial. Bone Joint J 2017;99-B(11):1520–5.

23. Hood MA, Murtha YM, Della Rocca GJ, et al. Prevalence of low vitamin D levels in patients with orthopedic trauma. Am J Orthop (Belle Mead NJ) 2016;45(7):E522–6.

24. Sprague S, Bhandari M, Devji T, et al. Prescription of vitamin D to fracture patients: a lack of consensus and evidence. J Orthop Trauma 2016; 30(2):e64–9.

25. Schiffman B, Summers H, Bernstein M, et al. Hypovitaminosis D in orthopaedic trauma: which guidelines should be followed? J Orthop Trauma 2018; 32(8):e295–9.

26. Andres BA, Childs BR, Vallier HA. Treatment of hypovitaminosis D in an orthopaedic trauma population. J Orthop Trauma 2018;32(4): e129–33.

27. U.S. Department of Health and Human Services and U.S. Department of Agriculture. Dietary guidelines for Americans 2015-2020 2015. Available at: https://health.gov/dietaryguidelines/2015/guidelines/. Accessed October 1, 2018.

28. Hoel DG, Berwick M, de Gruijl FR, et al. The risks and benefits of sun exposure 2016. Dermatoendocrinol 2016;8(1):e1248325.

29. Final recommendation statement: vitamin D and calcium to prevent fractures: preventive medication. U.S. Preventive Services Task Force. Available at: https://www.uspreventiveservicestaskforce. org/Page/Document/RecommendationStatement-Final/vitamin-d-and-calcium-to-prevent-fractures-preventive-medication. Accessed October 1, 2018.

30. Jones G. Pharmacokinetics of vitamin D toxicity. Am J Clin Nutr 2008;88(2):582S–6S.
31. National Institutes of Health: office of dietary supplements. Calcium fact sheet for health professionals. Available at: https://ods.od.nih.gov/factsheets/Calcium-HealthProfessional/. Accessed October 1, 2018.
32. Kenny AM, Prestwood KM, Biskup B, et al. Comparison of the effects of calcium loading with calcium citrate or calcium carbonate on bone turnover in postmenopausal women. Osteoporos Int 2004; 15(4):290–4.
33. Sakhaee K, Bhuket T, Adams-Huet B, et al. Meta-analysis of calcium bioavailability: a comparison of calcium citrate with calcium carbonate. Am J Ther 1999;6(6):313–21.
34. Domrongkitchaiporn S, Ongphiphadhanakul B, Stitchantrakul W, et al. Risk of calcium oxalate nephrolithiasis in postmenopausal women supplemented with calcium or combined calcium and estrogen. Maturitas 2002;41(2):149–56.
35. Lee NK, Sowa H, Hinoi E, et al. Endocrine regulation of energy metabolism by the skeleton. Cell 2007;130(3):456–69.
36. Palermo A, Tuccinardi D, D'Onofrio L, et al. Vitamin K and osteoporosis: myth or reality? Metabolism 2017;70:57–71.
37. Gage BF, Birman-Deych E, Radford MJ, et al. Risk of osteoporotic fracture in elderly patients taking warfarin: results from the National Registry of Atrial Fibrillation 2. Arch Intern Med 2006; 166(2):241–6.
38. Namba S, Yamaoka-Tojo M, Hashikata T, et al. Long-term warfarin therapy and biomarkers for osteoporosis and atherosclerosis. BBA Clin 2015; 4:76–80.
39. Haas AV, LeBoff MS. Osteoanabolic agents for osteoporosis. J Endocr Soc 2018;2(8):922–32.
40. Varela A, Chouinard L, Lesage E, et al. One year of abaloparatide, a selective peptide activator of the PTH1 receptor, increased bone mass and strength in ovariectomized rats. Bone 2017;95:143–50.
41. Cosman F, Hattersley G, Hu MY, et al. Effects of abaloparatide-sc on fractures and bone mineral density in subgroups of postmenopausal women with osteoporosis and varying baseline risk factors. J Bone Miner Res 2017;32(1):17–23.
42. Giannotti S, Bottai V, Dell'Osso G, et al. Atrophic femoral nonunion successfully treated with teriparatide. Eur J Orthop Surg Traumatol 2013; 23(Suppl 2):S291–4.
43. Lee YK, Ha YC, Koo KH. Teriparatide, a nonsurgical solution for femoral nonunion? A report of three cases. Osteoporos Int 2012;23(12):2897–900.

Pediatrics

The Role of Vitamin D in Pediatric Orthopedics

Michael P. Horan, MD, MS[a,*], Kevin Williams, MD[b], Daniel Hughes, PhD[b]

KEYWORDS

• Vitamin D • Pediatric orthopedics • Rickets • Deficiency • Fracture risk • Calcium • Phosphate

---

KEY POINTS

- Understanding the role of vitamin D is an important component of the proper care of the pediatric orthopedic patient.
- Vitamin D is an essential component of bone metabolism in the growth and development of the pediatric skeleton, which can be acutely affected by changes to the body's vitamin D, calcium, and phosphate levels, resulting in pathologic conditions such as rickets or fractures.
- This article reviews the main areas in which vitamin D relates to pediatric orthopedics and highlights some of the areas where future research is being directed.

INTRODUCTION

For the pediatric orthopedic surgeon, understanding the role of vitamin D is an important component of the proper care of the pediatric orthopedic patient. Vitamin D is an essential component of bone metabolism in the growth and development of the pediatric skeleton. Bone homeostasis can be acutely affected by changes to the body's vitamin D, calcium, and phosphate levels, resulting in pathologic conditions such as vitamin D–dependent rickets, osteoporosis, and a predisposition to fractures. This article reviews the main areas in which vitamin D relates to pediatric orthopedics and highlights some of the areas where future research is being directed.

VITAMIN D: WHAT'S ALL THE RECENT FUSS?

Within the last decade, multiple studies have demonstrated the potential health benefits of vitamin D supplementation, including improved bone health, reduced fracture risk, protection from autoimmune disease, and decreased cancer risk.[1,2] A review of the Medline database from the 1950s through 2017 shows that the number of studies related to both vitamin D and pediatric orthopedics has been exponentially increasing over the past 20 years (**Fig. 1**).[3] The intensified recognition of the role of vitamin D has therefore become an area of concern as modern dietary and lifestyle changes affect both the intake and production of vitamin D. As such, a recent study has demonstrated that the number of US adults taking vitamin D supplements has increased significantly over the past 2 decades.[4]

Vitamin D deficiency is also a common concern in pediatric populations, significantly affecting at-risk populations such as non-white patients, obese patients, and patients with chronic illnesses such as cystic fibrosis and chronic kidney disease.[5] This finding is especially troubling because the percentage of obese children is increasing.[6] Additionally, a poor diet and minimal sun exposure increase a child's risk of vitamin D deficiency.[7] According to the American Academy of Orthopedic Surgeons, there

---

Disclosure Statement: Neither authors have any financial or related disclosures relevant to the material presented in this article.

[a] Pediatric Orthopaedic Surgery, Palmetto Health-USC Orthopaedic Center, University of South Carolina, 14 Medical Park, Suite 200, Columbia, SC 29203, USA; [b] Department of Orthopaedic Surgery, University of South Carolina School of Medicine, Medical Park 2, Suite 400, Columbia, SC 29203, USA

* Corresponding author.

E-mail address: michael.horan@palmettohealth.org

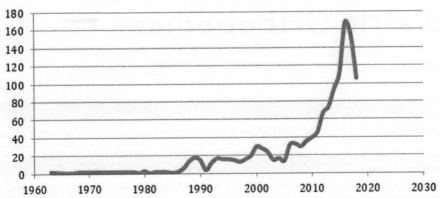

Fig. 1. Number of Indexed Research articles vs Year 1960-2018. *Data from* Alexandru Dan Corlan. Medline trend: automated yearly statistics of PubMed results for any query, 2004. Web resource at URL: http://dan.corlan.net/medline-trend.html. Accessed: 2012-02-14. (Archived by WebCite at http://www.webcitation.org/65RkD48SV).

are not a significant number of foods that contain high doses of vitamin D, so even the healthiest of diets may not include enough.[8] Children frequently spend more time indoors using computers, which affects their ability to synthesize vitamin D. Newer arguments have emerged that use of sunscreens has had an unintended[9–16] effect on decreased vitamin D synthesis. There remains debate as to the usefulness of vitamin D monitoring, acceptable serum levels, and their relation to clinical practice.[15,17–24]

VITAMIN D: HISTORICAL PERSPECTIVE

The discovery of vitamin D as a component of the calcium–phosphate regulation pathway came out of investigations into the causes of rickets, which plagued children in the late part of the 19th and early part of the 20th century. Deluca,[25] Zhang and colleagues,[26] and Holick[27] provide a thorough and interesting review of this history dating back to 1645. The critical time for vitamin D discovery comes just after the exploding studies into vital amines, or vitamins, discovered by Casimir Funk in 1912.[28] In1919, Sir Edward Mellanby discovered vitamin D and its role in rickets.[26] The relationship between the lack of sunlight exposure in industrialized England along with the observation of the preventative effects of the folk remedy of cod liver oil lead to this discovery. Elmer McCollum was another important researcher in the United States who helped to discover vitamins A and B, and while doing so theorized about the existence of another substance protecting against rickets. Kurt Huldschinsky of Germany made the association of UV light exposure and improvement of clinical rickets. Both UV light

and cod liver oil's curative action for rickets lead to the discovery of vitamin D's role in calcium-phosphate regulation.[25,29] Since that time, the relationship between vitamin D, calcium, and phosphate has continued to be investigated leading to new discoveries of vitamin D's role in bone health, infections, cancer prevention, asthma and allergies, and neurologic development.[1,2,30–38]

VITAMIN D–CALCIUM–PHOSPHATE PATHWAY REVIEW

Vitamin D regulation of calcium and phosphate is a complex process involving multiple organs and receptors in the body. The details of this pathway are well-documented in multiple sources and are available for review.[27,39–41] In brief, vitamin D takes 2 active forms, vitamin D_2 and vitamin D_3. Vitamin D_2 is created in plants and is called ergocalciferol. The other active form is vitamin D_3 (cholecalciferol), which is synthesized through a pathway directed initially by the skin. Both active forms can also be found in nutritional supplements of several varieties and dosages, usually described in international units (IU).

The human vitamin D_3 synthesis pathway starts in the dermal layer of the skin where 7-dehydrocholesterol is converted to cholecalciferol/vitamin D_3 via UV radiation stimulus. The liver then plays a role by adding a hydroxyl group to create 25(OH)-vitamin D3, which is converted to 1,25(OH)$_2$ vitamin D_3 via its renal pathway. This remains as its active form. This simplified pathway is outlined in **Fig. 2**. The active form of vitamin D effects osteoclastic release and intestinal adsorption of calcium and phosphate. Further, vitamin D influences renal control of reabsorption or excretion

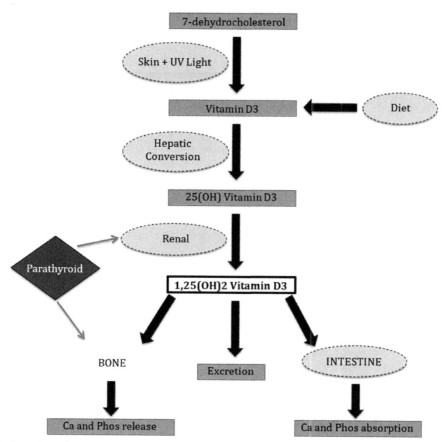

Fig. 2. Basic pathway for Vitamin D synthesis and calcium-phosphate regulation. Ca and Phos, calcium and phosphorous in serum. (*Data from* Feldman D, editor. Vitamin D, volume I: biochemistry, physiology and diagnostics. 4th edition. London: Elsevier; 2018.)

or the 2 minerals. The genes that code for the receptors and enzymes that control this signaling process are the basis for the genetic causes of hereditary rickets, as discussed elsewhere in this article. Several feedback loops exist to decrease release of the active form of vitamin D_3, which include serum parathyroid levels, as well as the calcium and phosphate levels themselves. The role of parathyroid hormone in the regulation of these levels is also the basis for the metabolic effects of primary and secondary hyperparathyroidism (seen with dietary deficiencies) and associated disorders hypoparathyroidism and pseudohypoparathyroidism.

Dietary regulation of calcium homeostasis is the primary role of vitamin D in its active form. Vitamin D increases dietary uptake of calcium in the gut via modulation of transcription factors and also activates osteoclastic resorption of bone, which releases calcium, creating an increase in overall calcium and phosphate levels in the bloodstream.

PEDIATRIC ORTHOPEDIC WORKUP

Abnormal calcium and phosphate homeostasis can be due to multiple etiologies. A general pediatric workup includes a detailed history and physical to identify any historical factors consistent with any conditions predisposing to deficiency of vitamin D or consistent with familial vitamin D abnormalities. In addition to the family medical history, a thorough dietary evaluation pinpoints issues with gastrointestinal uptake of calcium and phosphate. Past surgical, medical, fracture, and medication history should also be obtained. Concurrently, a physical examination always precludes any laboratory or radiographic workup. Given the intricacies and involvement of multiple metabolic pathways within musculoskeletal homeostasis, several laboratory markers should be obtained simultaneously as vitamin D if any abnormalities are suspected. A suggested basic bone metabolic workup might include laboratory analysis of 25(OH)vitamin D, serum calcium, serum phosphate, parathyroid hormone, and alkaline phosphatase. Laboratory relations to common causes of disruption in calcium and vitamin D normalization are listed in Table 1, but it is recommended for specialist referral if findings other than dietary deficiency are noted to elucidate the cause of the abnormal laboratory findings. More detailed inspection of ionized calcium, albumin levels or blood protein levels, and tests for vitamin D precursors are best interpreted by an endocrinologist or bone metabolic specialist.

VITAMIN D DEFICIENCY

Vitamin D deficiency is a global concern in both the pediatric and the adult setting. It is most commonly found in Asia and in zones of lower economic status. Estimates for the rate of vitamin D deficiency in the United States range from 30% to 70%.[42,43] Fig. 3 illustrates the distribution of estimated pediatric vitamin D deficiency worldwide.[43] The focus of this article is on pediatric orthopedics and vitamin D; however, the skeletal manifestations of vitamin D deficiency have been termed only the "tip of the vitamin D iceberg"[27] owing to the possible effects of developing other chronic diseases including multiple sclerosis, diabetes, psychiatric conditions, and disorders of immunomodulation.

Determining what constitutes a deficiency of vitamin D depends on which reference a clinician uses. Vitamin D has been described classically as being deficient, normal, or toxic based on serum 25-hydroxyvitamin D [25(OH)D] levels.[15] More recently however, various groups have categorized vitamin D status as being either sufficient or deficient.[44–46] Some authors offer 3 categories: deficient, insufficient, or sufficient.[24,47,48]

This is tabulated in Table 2 as a way of showing the potential confusion from multiple different standards. Further confusion can result from some authors using the alternative units of nmol/L or even using other names for 25(OH)D including calcifediol or calcidiol.[49] These different resources and make it difficult to determine a patient's true vitamin D status. This discrepancy could lead to the undertreatment of some at-risk pediatric populations. The most commonly used source is that of the Endocrine Society's[44,47] definition of deficiency at less than 20 ng/mL, insufficiency at 30 ng/mL or less, and sufficiency at greater than 30 ng/mL. In 2015,[50] a comparative cohort study showed that 58 pediatric patients with low-energy fractures had similar 25(OH)D serum levels as pediatric patients with chronic kidney disease (27.5 ng/mL vs 24.6 ng/mL, respectively).[50] They show that using a cutoff of 32 ng/mL for vitamin D insufficiency may be more appropriate for children with fractures because it will reveal a larger percentage of the children needing vitamin D supplementation, which should decrease risk for low-energy fractures. There are several reviews published on the topic of treatment of vitamin D deficiency[5,19,45,47,49,51,52] that provide additional resources of information on the topic.

In vitamin D deficiency, a small portion of calcium (10%–15%) and phosphorous (50%–60%) are absorbed from the diet.[27] This state causes parathyroid hormone release, which acts on bone to release calcium as well as the kidney, which decreases renal wasting of calcium and increases excretion of phosphorus.[27] These changes to the calcium and phosphorous balance are what lead to the decreased boney mineralization seen in nutritional rickets.

Table 1
Basic laboratory findings in vitamin D, calcium, and phosphate metabolism

Disease Process	Serum Calcium	Serum Phosphate	PTH	Alkaline Phosphatase	25(OH) Vitamin D
Nutritional rickets	↓ or ↔	↓	↑	↑	↓
Vitamin D dependent: type I[a]	↓	↓	↑	↑	↔
Vitamin D dependent: type II[a]	↓	↓	↑	↑	↔
Vitamin D-resistant rickets[b] (hypophosphatemic)	↔	↓	↔	↑	↔

Abbreviations: ↓, value lower than normal; ↑, value higher than normal; ↔, normal; PTH, parathyroid hormone.
[a] Additional laboratory analysis needed to differentiate between these types.
[b] X-linked, autosomal-dominant and recessive forms need additional workup by subspecialist.
Data from Refs.[18,27,41,65]

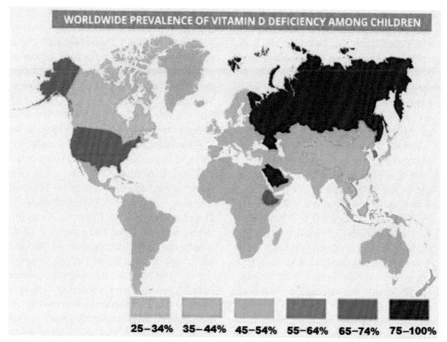

Fig. 3. Worldwide distribution of vitamin D deficiency. (*From* Tovey A, Cannell JJ. High prevalence of vitamin D deficiency among children worldwide. The vitamin D council blog & newsletter, 3/2017. Available at: https://www.vitamindcouncil.org/high-prevalence-of-vitamin-d-deficiency-among-children-worldwide/. Accessed October 29, 2018; with permission.)

Risk factors, such as hyperpigmentation, reduced sun exposure, seasonal affects, older age, and obesity, are important for screening the potential need for vitamin D deficiency.[49,53–55] In a study from 2016,[53] 52% of patients with a fracture that had at least 1 of these 3 risk factors were also vitamin D deficient (25(OH)D <20 ng/mL). Race may play a role, but this difference could be related to one of the aforementioned factors.[23,56]

In terms of prevention of vitamin D deficiency, multiple reviews and consensus opinions have been publish on the topic including an interesting study on photobiology using the vitamin D levels of a tribe in Tanzania that still uses primitive hunter gatherer lifestyle to establish a baseline human normal serum value owing to evolutionary sun exposure, then calculates an equivalent oral supplementation value associated with that sun exposure. For adults, this was calculated to be 2000 IU of vitamin D_3 daily.[57] The resource most widely used is the Institute of Medicine 2011 publication "Dietary Reference Intakes (DRI) for Calcium and Vitamin

Table 2
Differing levels and characterizations of vitamin D deficiency examples, 2010-2018

	Severely Deficient	Deficient	Insufficient	Sufficient
Polish Society of Pediatric Endocrinology and Diabetes (2018)[48]	<10	<20	20–30	>30
Italian Pediatric Society (2018)[24]	<10	<20	20–30	>30
Global Consensus (2016)[46]	—	<12	12–20	>20
The Endocrine Society (2011)[47]	—	<20	20–30	>30
Pediatric Endocrine Society (2011)[45]	≤5	≤15	15–20	>20
Institute of Medicine (2010)[44]	—	<12	12–20	>20

D,"[44] which encompassed a systematic review of published studies as well as data from the US National Health and Nutrition Examination Survey. These DRIs were intended to be applicable to the North American population, excluding patients with rare diseases but including those with conditions considered to be widespread such as obesity. Their recommendation was for 400 IU of vitamin D for infants ages 0 to 12 months and a 600 IU of vitamin D for children ages 1 to 18 years. These values are listed in **Table 2**.

In 2011, the Endocrine Society[47] released a recommendation for individuals at risk of vitamin D deficiency of a daily requirement of 400 to 1000 IU of vitamin D for infants ages 0 to 12 months and a 600 to 1000 IU of vitamin D for children ages 1 to 18 years. Although these daily requirement recommendations have remain unchanged, the optimum functional serum circulating 25(OH)D level for pediatric patients remains widely disputed.[16,23,24,38,39,44–48,58,59]

Along with vitamin D recommendations, oral intake of calcium is also vitally important. The same Institute of Medicine publication presented recommendations for calcium intake for children as well. These values are also listed in **Table 2**.

VITAMIN D–ASSOCIATED BONY PATHOLOGY

Various pathologies are associated with vitamin D deficiency. There is the well-known association with bone health, evidenced by the historical discovery of vitamin D through investigations into the causes and treatments of rickets. The origin of the term rickets itself is unclear, possibly stemming from the German word *wricken*, meaning twisted[60,61] or from the Greek word *rachitis*, referring to the effects on the spine.[29] Rickets has been classically defined as the failure to mineralize new bone formation,[60] the result of which causes altered bone growth owing to the abnormal mineralization, commonly leading to widening of the physis and cupping of the metaphysis. This leads to bowing of the long bones as well as the classic rachitic rosary appearance of the cupped or flared ends of the ribs. The most common form of rickets has always been what has been referred to as nutritional rickets. The incidence and prevalence of nutritional rickets had significantly decreased in the 20th century as nutritional treatments were developed; however, a 2014 study in *The Lancet*[62] noted that rates of admission to hospitals for rickets related conditions were at their highest in the last 5 decades. Similar studies in Scotland

have shown increases as well.[63] In the United States, rates have also been increasing.[64] Reasons for this were hypothesized to include an actual increase in disease prevalence, and possible increased coding and documentation practices, diagnostics, or admission standards. The actual reasons are yet to be elucidated, but are felt to be more likely related to disease process instead of the other factors listed.[62]

Besides classic nutritional rickets, other forms of rickets include vitamin D-dependent rickets, vitamin D-resistant rickets, and then those from other causes such as chronic kidney disease, or renal osteodystrophy.[65] Vitamin D-dependent rickets (types 1, 2 and 3), are characterized by inherited gene mutations that affect the renal conversion to the active form of vitamin D or a defect in the vitamin D receptor or the vitamin D receptor element complex.[27,65] Vitamin D-resistant rickets (X-linked familial hypophosphatemic rickets, autosomal-dominant hypophosphatemic rickets, and tumor-induced rickets) all involve an increase in the amount of fibroblast growth factor 23, which allows renal wasting of phosphate, resulting in hypophosphatemia.[27,65]

The treatment for the various forms and causes of rickets begins first with the proper diagnosis. Often it is the pediatric orthopedist who evaluates a patient with a presentation concerning for rickets owing to referral for leg alignment concerns or other deformity. The help of endocrinology experts in the interpretation of the detailed studies on vitamin D precursors and errors in the calcium–phosphate regulatory pathway typically augments the work up of a rickettsial patient. Each of these forms of rickets needs a team approach to treatment, including proper diagnosis, nutritional management, or medicine administration of the appropriate precursor or metabolite before surgical management. Primary care (pediatrics/family medicine) and specialists including an endocrinologist and geneticist, as well as ancillary experts in nutrition are often needed to help in producing a proper diagnosis and satisfactory outcomes for the patient and physician. The specific medical and surgical treatments for rickets are beyond the scope of this review.

VITAMIN D AND FRACTURE RISK

In addition to bone formation, bone healing is also an important factor that may be related to vitamin D status. It has long been theorized that vitamin D deficiency is related to increased fracture risk and this topic has been evaluated with multiple studies. In the consensus study document "Global Consensus Recommendations on Prevention and Management of Nutritional Rickets,"[46] an expert group reviewed evidence-based studies to determine recommendations related to prevention of nutritional rickets. As part of the review, it was stated based on observational studies and case reports that children with radiographically confirmed rickets have an increased risk of fracture and that children with simple vitamin D deficiency are not at increased risk of fracture. This was given a value of a strong recommendation with levels of evidence were deemed to be of a moderate quality.[46] Since that consensus, there have been a host of studies looking into the relationship between vitamin D and fracture risk with mixed findings (**Table 3**).

In support of the findings outlined in the global consensus statement, a study of emergency room patients from 2014[66] showed that there was no difference between vitamin D levels in 100 children under the age of 18 who had a fracture versus those who did not. Recently, Minkowitz and colleagues[67] found no increased fracture risk associated with vitamin D level; however, they did find a higher risk of more severe fracture with lower vitamin D value. In 2008, Olney and colleagues[22] looked at a variety of metabolic factors and found an association between frequent fracture and hypercalciuria, but did not find a significant number of patients with vitamin D deficiency in the population of fracture patients and controls in a Northern Florida population. A report from Anderson and colleagues[68] in 2017 showed no correlation between vitamin D levels and fracture risk, but did find that children who were given vitamin D supplements by their parent had a lower risk for fractures. A 2018 Polish study[69,70] did not have enough cases to correlate vitamin D and fracture risk but did show alternatively that lower vitamin K levels were correlation with increased fracture risk.

Contrary to the findings discussed, a 2017 study showed that children with fractures had significantly lower 25(OH)D as compared with normal children (14.5 ng/mL vs 21.3 ng/mL).[71] Similarly, an Egyptian study showed an increased rate of vitamin D deficiency and decreased bone mineral density in children with forearm fractures in 2016.[72] Findings in Australia of the same nature were noted by Kwon and colleagues[53] in 2016.

Most of the studies on fractures and vitamin D deficiency have been published in the years since the Global Consensus[46] stated their findings that there was a "strong recommendation and moderate evidence" to suggest that vitamin D deficiency does not contribute to fracture risk

Table 3
Summary of findings from recent studies on vitamin D levels and pediatric fractures

Study	Findings	Comments
Contreras et al,[66] 2014	No difference	No difference in the proportions of sufficiency, insufficiency, or deficiency between groups
Minkowitz et al,[67] 2017	No difference	Lower vitamin D found in more severe fractures
Olney et al,[22] 2008	No difference	Association between hypercalciuria and increased fractures noted; low rate of vitamin D deficiency in study population
Anderson et al,[68] 2017	No difference	Lower risk of fractures in patients who received vitamin D supplements
Karpinski et al,[69] 2017	Not able to determine	Lower vitamin K levels correlated with an increased fracture risk
Saglam et al,[71] 2017	Lower vitamin D in pediatric fracture patients	Both groups were found to be below accepted values for "sufficiency"
El-Sakka et al,[72] 2016	Lower Vitamin D in pediatric fracture patients	Study on forearm fractures
Kwon et al,[53] 2016	Lower vitamin D in pediatric fracture patients	One-third of all participants classified as vitamin D deficient

outside the setting of nutritional rickets. The studies that have been presented illustrate conflicting results on the topic and additional well-designed studies that encompass large patient populations in multiple geographic areas are needed to encompass today's changing lifestyles, obesity rates, and decreased sun exposure.

NEW RESEARCH AREAS IN VITAMIN D AND PEDIATRIC ORTHOPEDICS

Additional areas of research and debate include postoperative healing, infection association,[73] role in Blount disease,[74,75] slipped capital femoral epiphysis,[34,35,76] and osteochondritis dissecans,[36] as well as association with muscle aches and pains.[30] A metaanalysis of infections and vitamin D supplementation in children under 5 years of age found no strong correlations between the mean serum vitamin D concentration in relation to either mortality, pneumonia index, diarrhea incidence, or hospitalization.[73] In 2 studies of vitamin D in Blount disease with obesity, 1 study found no differences in serum vitamin D status between the children with Blount disease versus the normal children.[74] The second study found that obese children with concomitant vitamin D deficiency (<16 ng/mL) had a positive association with Blount disease.[75] In relation to slipped capital femoral epiphysis (SCFE), 15 cases of SCFE in India were correlated with a higher body mass index and a lower serum vitamin D level (11.8 ng/mL) as compared with the controls (27.1 ng/mL).[35] A case study showing an obese child with SCFE and vitamin D deficiency was well-aided in their SCFE healing with vitamin D supplementation.[76] Furthermore, SCFE has been suggested to be more prevalent at longitudes above 35° North and between 31° and 35° North, which suggests a role of sun exposure and vitamin D production.[34] In a study of 80 juvenile patients with osteochondrosis dissecans between 2010 and 2015, the patients with osteochondrosis dissecans had lower vitamin D serum levels as compared with the control group, suggesting a role for vitamin D in the etiology of osteochondrosis dissecans.[36] In a Serbian study, 35 children with both vitamin D deficiency and a musculoskeletal or orthopedic condition were given vitamin D supplementation for 6 months and the child and parent-reported scores relating to pain decreased during this time.[30] There is only isolated research into these topics and the reader is encouraged to evaluate these for relevance and possible areas of further research.

VITAMIN D IN PEDIATRIC ORTHOPEDICS: PUTTING IT ALL TOGETHER

Vitamin D is well-established as a key component in the regulation of calcium, phosphate, and subsequent bone health. This connection was initially established during the investigations on rickets in the early part of the 20th century. Although there is a general consensus on the amount of vitamin D, it takes to prevent the formation of rickets,[44] what is unknown is how to best define vitamin D deficiency, and therefore the subsequent possible effect on fracture risk, bone healing, and extraskeletal benefits. At present, no major medical organization endorses population-wide screening for low vitamin D.[77] The biologic influence of low vitamin D levels and the health benefit of maintaining high serum 25(OH)D levels has not been established for the general population,[15] nor more specifically for the pediatric population. For the pediatric orthopedic practitioner, vitamin D is one of the most important vitamins involved in the homeostasis of the skeleton and those who provide care for children and their musculoskeletal health should be well aware of its mechanism and roles in bone health.[77,78] Future well-designed pediatric research studies that encompass multiple geographic and socioeconomic groups are needed to determine the effects of vitamin D levels on bone health outside of the known rickettsial associations. This research will help to educate all of us in the field of pediatric orthopedics and ultimately help to provide better care for our patients.

REFERENCES

1. Holick MF, Chen TC. Vitamin D deficiency: a worldwide problem with health consequences. Am J Clin Nutr 2008;87(4):1080S–6S.

2. Lappe JM, Travers-Gustafson D, Davies KM, et al. Vitamin D and calcium supplementation reduces cancer risk: results of a randomized trial. Am J Clin Nutr 2007;85(6):1586–91.

3. Corlan AD. Medline trend: automated yearly statistics of PubMed results for any query. Secondary Medline trend: automated yearly statistics of PubMed results for any query 2004. Available at: http://dan.corlan.net/medline-trend.html. Accessed August 15, 2018.

4. Rooney MR, Harnack L, Michos ED, et al. Trends in use of high-dose vitamin D supplements exceeding 1000 or 4000 international units daily, 1999-2014. JAMA 2017;317(23):2448–50.

5. Lee JY, So TY, Thackray J. A review on vitamin d deficiency treatment in pediatric patients. J Pediatr Pharmacol Ther 2013;18(4):277–91.

6. Cheng L. The convergence of two epidemics: vitamin D deficiency in obese school-aged children. J Pediatr Nurs 2018;38:20–6.

7. Ganji V, Martineau B, Van Fleit WE. Association of serum vitamin D concentrations with dietary patterns in children and adolescents. Nutr J 2018;17(1):58.

8. American Academy of Orthopaedic Surgeons. Vitamin D for good bone health. Secondary vitamin D for good bone health 2016. Available at: https://orthoinfo.aaos.org/en/staying-healthy/vitamin-d-for-good-bone-health/.

9. Abu-Abed A, Azbarga S, Peleg R. Knowledge and attitudes of family doctors, dermatologists, and endocrinologists on sun exposure and vitamin D. Postgrad Med 2018;130(5):477–80.

10. Bora NS, Mazumder B, Chattopadhyay P. Prospects of topical protection from ultraviolet radiation exposure: a critical review on the juxtaposition of the benefits and risks involved with the use of chemoprotective agents. J Dermatolog Treat 2018; 29(3):256–68.

11. Holick MF. Reply to Whiteman et al.: in-deed wise to get some sensible sun exposure. Br J Dermatol 2017;177(4):1136–7.

12. Holman DM, Berkowitz Z, Guy GP Jr, et al. The association between beliefs about vitamin D and skin cancer risk-related behaviors. Prev Med 2017;99: 326–31.

13. Libon F, Courtois J, Le Goff C, et al. Sunscreens block cutaneous vitamin D production with only a minimal effect on circulating 25-hydroxyvitamin D. Arch Osteoporos 2017;12(1):66.

14. Littlewood Z, Greenfield S. Parents' knowledge, attitudes and beliefs regarding sun protection in children: a qualitative study. BMC Public Health 2018; 18(1):207.

15. Reddy KK, Gilchrest BA. What is all this commotion about vitamin D? J Invest Dermatol 2010;130(2): 321–6.

16. American Academy of Dermatology. Position statement on vitamin D. Secondary position statement on vitamin D 2009. https://www.aad.org/forms/policies/uploads/ps/aad_ps_vitamin_d.pdf. Accessed August 15, 2018.

17. Clarke NM, Page JE. Vitamin D deficiency: a paediatric orthopaedic perspective. Curr Opin Pediatr 2012;24(1):46–9.

18. Dirks NF, Ackermans MT, Lips P, et al. The when, what & how of measuring vitamin D metabolism in clinical medicine. Nutrients 2018;10(4) [pii: E482].

19. Gartner LM, Greer FR. Prevention of rickets and vitamin D deficiency: new guidelines for vitamin D intake. Pediatrics 2003;111(4 Pt 1):908–10.

20. Iyer P, Diamond F. Detecting disorders of vitamin D deficiency in children: an update. Adv Pediatr 2013; 60(1):89–106.

21. Lawson DE. Dietary vitamin D: is it necessary? J Hum Nutr 1981;35(1):61–3.

22. Olney RC, Mazur JM, Pike LM, et al. Healthy children with frequent fractures: how much evaluation is needed? Pediatrics 2008;121(5):890–7.

23. Parry J, Sullivan E, Scott AC. Vitamin D sufficiency screening in preoperative pediatric orthopaedic patients. J Pediatr Orthop 2011;31(3):331–3.

24. Saggese G, Vierucci F, Prodam F, et al. Vitamin D in pediatric age: consensus of the Italian Pediatric Society and the Italian Society of Preventive and Social Pediatrics, jointly with the Italian Federation of Pediatricians. Ital J Pediatr 2018; 44(1):51.

25. Deluca HF. Historical overview of vitamin D. In: Feldman D, editor. Vitamin D, Volume I: biochemistry, physiology and diagnostics. 4th edition. San Diego (CA): Academic Press; 2018. p. 4–9.

26. Zhang M, Shen F, Petryk A, et al. "English disease": historical notes on rickets, the bone-lung link and child neglect issues. Nutrients 2016;8(11) [pii:E722].

27. Holick MF. Resurrection of vitamin D deficiency and rickets. J Clin Invest 2006;116(8):2062–72.

28. Rosenfeld L. Vitamine–vitamin. The early years of discovery. Clin Chem 1997;43(4):680–5.

29. O/'Riordan JLH, Bijvoet OLM. Rickets before the discovery of vitamin D. Bonekey Rep 2014;3:478.

30. Blagojevic Z, Nikolic V, Kisic-Tepavcevic D, et al. Musculoskeletal pain and vitamin D deficiency in children: a pilot follow-up study of vitamin D therapy in musculoskeletal/orthopedic conditions. Acta Chir Orthop Traumatol Cech 2016;83(1):21–6.

31. Brenckmann C, Papaioannou A. Bisphosphonates for osteoporosis in people with cystic fibrosis. Cochrane Database Syst Rev 2001;(4):CD002010.

32. Ferguson JH, Chang AB. Vitamin D supplementation for cystic fibrosis. Cochrane Database Syst Rev 2012;(4):CD007298.

33. Fluss J, Kern I, de Coulon G, et al. Vitamin D deficiency: a forgotten treatable cause of motor delay and proximal myopathy. Brain Dev 2014;36(1):84–7.

34. Loder RT, Schneble CA. Seasonal variation in slipped capital femoral epiphysis: new findings using a National Children's Hospital database. J Pediatr Orthop 2017. https://doi.org/10.1097/bpo.0000000000001074.

35. Madhuri V, Arora SK, Dutt V. Slipped capital femoral epiphysis associated with vitamin D deficiency: a series of 15 cases. Bone Joint J 2013;95-b(6):851–4.

36. Maier GS, Lazovic D, Maus U, et al. Vitamin D deficiency: the missing etiological factor in the development of juvenile osteochondrosis dissecans? J Pediatr Orthop 2016. https://doi.org/10.1097/bpo.0000000000000921.

37. Martineau AR, Cates CJ, Urashima M, et al. Vitamin D for the management of asthma. Cochrane Database Syst Rev 2016;(9):CD011511.

38. Paterson C. Vitamin D deficiency: a diagnosis often missed. Br J Hosp Med (Lond) 2011;72(8):456–8, 460–2.

39. Tran EY, Uhl RL, Rosenbaum AJ. Vitamin D in orthopaedics. JBJS Rev 2017;5(8):e1.

40. Patton CM, Powell AP, Patel AA. Vitamin D in orthopaedics. J Am Acad Orthop Surg 2012;20(3):123–9.

41. Vaishya R, Vijay V, Agarwal AK, et al. Resurgence of vitamin D: old wine in new bottle. J Clin Orthop Trauma 2015;6(3):173–83.

42. Kumar J, Muntner P, Kaskel FJ, et al. Prevalence and associations of 25-hydroxyvitamin D deficiency in US children: NHANES 2001-2004. Pediatrics 2009;124(3):e362–70.

43. Tovey AC, Cannell JJ. High prevalence of vitamin D deficiency among children worldwide. The Vitamin D Council Blog & Newsletter; 2017.

44. Ross AC, Taylor CL, Yaktine AL, editors. Dietary reference intakes for calcium and vitamin D. Washington, DC: National Academy of Sciences; 2011.

45. Misra M, Pacaud D, Petryk A, et al. Vitamin D deficiency in children and its management: review of current knowledge and recommendations. Pediatrics 2008;122(2):398–417.

46. Munns CF, Shaw N, Kiely M, et al. Global consensus recommendations on prevention and management of nutritional rickets. J Clin Endocrinol Metab 2016;101(2):394–415.

47. Holick MF, Binkley NC, Bischoff-Ferrari HA, et al. Evaluation, treatment, and prevention of vitamin D deficiency: an Endocrine Society clinical practice guideline. J Clin Endocrinol Metab 2011;96(7): 1911–30.

48. Rusinska A, Pludowski P, Walczak M, et al. Vitamin D supplementation guidelines for general population and groups at risk of Vitamin D deficiency in Poland: recommendations of the Polish Society of Pediatric Endocrinology and Diabetes and the Expert Panel with participation of National Specialist Consultants and representatives of scientific societies: 2018 update. Front Endocrinol (Lausanne) 2018;9:246.

49. Gorter EA, Oostdijk W, Felius A, et al. Vitamin D deficiency in pediatric fracture patients: prevalence, risk factors, and Vitamin D supplementation. J Clin Res Pediatr Endocrinol 2016;8(4):445–51.

50. Fabricant PD, Dy CJ, McLaren SH, et al. Low vitamin D levels in children with fractures: a comparative cohort study. HSS J 2015;11(3): 249–57.

51. Balasubramanian S, Dhanalakshmi K, Amperayani S. Vitamin D deficiency in childhood-a review of current guidelines on diagnosis and management. Indian Pediatr 2013;50(7):669–75.

52. Holick MF. The D-lightful vitamin D for child health. JPEN J Parenter Enteral Nutr 2012;36(1 Suppl): 9s–19s.

53. Kwon DH, Krieser D, Harris C, et al. High prevalence of vitamin D deficiency in 2-17 year olds presenting with acute fractures in southern Australia. Bone Rep 2016;5:153–7.

54. Thompson RM, Dean DM, Goldberg S, et al. Vitamin D insufficiency and fracture risk in urban children. J Pediatr Orthop 2017;37(6):368–73.

55. Wilsford LD, Sullivan E, Mazur LJ. Risk factors for vitamin D deficiency in children with osteogenesis imperfecta. J Pediatr Orthop 2013;33(5):575–9.

56. Ryan LM, Chamberlain JM, Singer SA, et al. Genetic influences on vitamin D status and forearm fracture risk in African American children. J Investig Med 2012;60(6):902–6.

57. Krzyscin JW, Guzikowski J, Rajewska-Wiech B. Optimal vitamin D3 daily intake of 2000IU inferred from modeled solar exposure of ancestral humans in Northern Tanzania. J Photochem Photobiol B 2016;159:101–5.

58. Casey CF, Slawson DC, Neal LR. Vitamin D supplementation in infants, children, and adolescents. Am Fam Physician 2010;81(6):745–8.

59. Winzenberg TM, Powell S, Shaw KA, et al. Vitamin D supplementation for improving bone mineral density in children. Cochrane Database Syst Rev 2010;(10):CD006944.

60. Elder CJ, Bishop NJ. Rickets. Lancet 2014; 383(9929):1665–76.

61. Hochberg Z. Rickets–past and present. Introduction. Endocr Dev 2003;6:1–13.

62. Goldacre M, Hall N, Yeates DG. Hospitalisation for children with rickets in England: a historical perspective. Lancet 2014;383(9917):597–8.

63. Ahmed SF, Franey C, McDevitt H, et al. Recent trends and clinical features of childhood vitamin D deficiency presenting to a children's hospital in Glasgow. Arch Dis Child 2011;96(7):694–6.

64. Kreiter SR, Schwartz RP, Kirkman HN Jr, et al. Nutritional rickets in African American breast-fed infants. J Pediatr 2000;137(2):153–7.

65. Nield LS, Mahajan P, Joshi A, et al. Rickets: not a disease of the past. Am Fam Physician 2006;74(4): 619–26.

66. Contreras JJ, Hiestand B, O'Neill JC, et al. Vitamin D deficiency in children with fractures. Pediatr Emerg Care 2014;30(11):777–81.

67. Minkowitz B, Cerame B, Poletick E, et al. Low Vitamin D levels are associated with need for surgical correction of pediatric fractures. J Pediatr Orthop 2017;37(1):23–9.

68. Anderson LN, Heong SW, Chen Y, et al. Vitamin D and fracture risk in early childhood: a case-control study. Am J Epidemiol 2017;185(12):1255–62.

69. Karpinski M, Popko J, Maresz K, et al. Roles of vitamins D and K, nutrition, and lifestyle in low-energy bone fractures in children and young adults. J Am Coll Nutr 2017;36(5):399–412.

70. Popko J, Karpiński M, Chojnowska S, et al. Decreased Levels of Circulating Carboxylated Osteocalcin in Children with Low Energy Fractures: A Pilot Study. Nutrients 2018;10(6).

71. Saglam Y, Kizildag H, Toprak G, et al. Prevalence of vitamin D insufficiency in children with forearm fractures. J Child Orthop 2017;11(3):180–4.

72. El-Sakka A, Penon C, Hegazy A, et al. Evaluating bone health in Egyptian children with forearm fractures: a case control study. Int J Pediatr 2016;2016: 7297092.

73. Yakoob MY, Salam RA, Khan FR, et al. Vitamin D supplementation for preventing infections in children under five years of age. Cochrane Database Syst Rev 2016;(11):CD008824.

74. Lisenda L, Simmons D, Firth GB, et al. Vitamin D status in blount disease. J Pediatr Orthop 2016; 36(5):e59–62.

75. Montgomery CO, Young KL, Austen M, et al. Increased risk of Blount disease in obese children and adolescents with vitamin D deficiency. J Pediatr Orthop 2010;30(8):879–82.

76. Skelley NW, Papp DF, Lee RJ, et al. Slipped capital femoral epiphysis with severe vitamin D deficiency. Orthopedics 2010;33(12):921.

77. Manson JE, Bassuk SS. Vitamin d research and clinical practice: at a crossroads. JAMA 2015;313(13): 1311–2.

78. Feldman D, Pike JW, Bouillon R. Vitamin D. 4th edition. London: Academic Press; 2018.

Osteogenesis Imperfecta
A Pediatric Orthopedic Perspective

Jeanne M. Franzone, MD[a],*, Suken A. Shah, MD[a],
Maegen J. Wallace, MD[b], Richard W. Kruse, DO, MBA[a]

KEYWORDS

- Osteogenesis imperfecta • Brittle bones • Extremity deformity • Spine deformity

KEY POINTS

- Osteogenesis imperfecta (OI) is a genetic connective tissue disorder characterized by low bone density, fractures, spine and extremity deformity, and several nonorthopedic manifestations.
- Medical management includes nutrition, adequate vitamin D and calcium intake, and activity and may include the use of bisphosphonates or other anabolic agents.
- Care should be managed by a cohesive multidisciplinary team.
- The orthopedic care of patients with OI includes fracture care and management of spine and extremity deformity with a goal of maximizing each individual's developmental and functional capacity.

BACKGROUND

Osteogenesis imperfecta (OI), also known as brittle bone disease, is a genetic connective tissue disorder characterized by low bone density, fractures, spine and extremity deformity for those with a severe form of the disease, and other extraskeletal manifestations.[1,2] It is genetically and phenotypically heterogeneous with a wide range of clinical severity.

The term osteogenesis imperfecta was coined by William Vrolik in the 1840s.[3,4] The widely used Sillence classification was initially described in 1979[5] and identified four primary types of OI:

    Type I: Mild, nondeforming
    Type II: Lethal perinatal
    Type III: Severe, progressively deforming
    Type IV: Phenotypically variable with white sclera

In the early 1980s, type I collagen mutations were first associated with autosomal-dominant OI.[6,7] The genes COL1A1 and COL1A2 code for type I collagen, which is a heterotrimer containing two α1 chains and one α2 chain that form a triple helix and is a significant component of the extracellular matrix in bone, helping to provide its strength. This may be likened to an analogy that type I collagen serves a role similar to that served by a reinforcing bar in concrete. An issue with the quality of type I collagen may cause a more moderate or severe form of OI, whereas an issue with the quantity of type I collagen may cause more mild forms of OI.[8] The disease severity may vary even among family members carrying the same mutation.

A clinically distinct form of OI, OI type V, was identified in Montreal with patients demonstrating calcification of the forearm interosseous membrane, hyperplastic callus, and an autosomal-dominant inheritance not associated with collagen type I mutations.[9] In 2006, a recessive form of lethal OI was reported to be caused by a mutation in CRTAP, a gene that encodes a

[a] Department of Orthopaedic Surgery, Nemours Alfred I. duPont Hospital for Children, 1600 Rockland Road, Wilmington, DE 19803, USA; [b] Department of Orthopaedic Surgery, University of Nebraska Medical Center, Children's Hospital and Medical Center, 8200 Dodge Street, Omaha, NE 68114, USA
* Corresponding author.
E-mail address: Jeanne.Franzone@nemours.org

Orthop Clin N Am 50 (2019) 193–209
https://doi.org/10.1016/j.ocl.2018.10.003
0030-5898/19/© 2018 Elsevier Inc. All rights reserved.

protein that plays a role in the post-translational modification of collagen.[8] The past decade has witnessed the recognition of an expanding number of recessive forms of OI responsible for approximately 15% of cases of OI caused by mutations in genes encoding proteins involved in the synthesis or processing of type I collagen. Some investigators have supported the creation of a new numbered type of OI associated with each of these genetic causes, with a list of 18 types and counting (Table 1).[2] Others have proposed a more clinically based approach in which each of the newly identified recessive types is incorporated into a clinical Sillence type based on the phenotypic presentation.[10] The designations of mild, moderate, and severe may also be used on a clinical basis. Although the diagnosis of OI is a clinical one, knowledge of the underlying genetic cause helps the pediatric orthopedist better understand the clinical characteristics and orthopedic phenotypes of the different forms of OI and enhance understanding of the responses to treatment and surgical intervention.

CLINICAL PRESENTATION AND CARE TEAM

Given the widespread role of type I collagen, there are a multitude of clinical manifestations of OI. The skeletal manifestations vary with disease severity and include low bone mass, fractures, bowing of the long bones in the extremities, vertebral compression fractures, basilar invagination, scoliosis, spondylolisthesis, ligamentous laxity, joint deformities, and short stature.[1] The extraskeletal manifestations may be present at birth or develop. These may include blue sclerae; hydrocephalus; hearing loss; dentinogenesis imperfecta; dental malocclusion; and pulmonary, cardiac, or gastrointestinal issues.

The management of OI, therefore, must involve a coordinated multidisciplinary care team with OI experience. As is the case with all diseases requiring complex multidisciplinary care, the coordination and communication among the care team is critical. Transition of care through adulthood plays an important role as young adults with OI take on the responsibility of their care at a time when they may be "aging out" of care in a pediatric environment.[11] Given the importance of multidisciplinary care of this complex condition, the transitional care of patients with OI is a focus of many large OI centers and the Osteogenesis Imperfecta Foundation.

CLINICAL MANAGEMENT

There is currently no cure for OI. Children are initially evaluated for the frequency of fractures and the presence of long bone deformity. Bone density may be part of the diagnostic evaluation and is also followed on a regular basis. The mainstays of the medical management of OI include nutrition and activity. Adequate amounts of calcium and vitamin D are essential for optimizing bone health in the setting of OI. Vitamin D and calcium levels must be followed as part of the medical management of patients with OI and supplementation doses adjusted accordingly.

Bisphosphonates are a class of antiresorptive drugs shown to increase bone mass, improve vertebral size and shape, and potentially reduce the frequency of fractures in patients with OI.[12–14] There is noted to be variability of the indications for bisphosphonate therapy and the dosing and the duration from center to center. A single vertebral body fracture is considered by many to be an indication for starting or resuming bisphosphonate therapy and three or more long bone fractures per year for 2 years. Anecdotally, bisphosphonates may help with bone pain. The results of yearly bone density (DEXA) scans may also play a role in the clinical decision making regarding the use of bisphosphonates.

Additional agents are currently being investigated in the setting of OI. Sclerostin antibody has been studied as an anabolic treatment approach and may have a synergistic effect when combined with a low-dose bisphosphonate.[15] Denosumab is a human monoclonal antibody that blocks RANKL, which is an essential cytokine in the osteoclastogenesis pathway and is currently being tested in patients with OI.[1] Cell therapy and gene targeting may play a role in the future, but are currently far from a clinical reality.

ORTHOPEDIC MANAGEMENT

The goal of the orthopedic management of children and adults with OI is to maximize function, achieve developmental milestones as close as possible to a child's peer group, and decrease deformity and fracture burden. Physical activity is an instrumental component of reaching this goal. Some form of activity, which may be tailored based on the disease severity, is important for everyone with OI to maximize functional ability. Although muscle strength is affected by OI, exercise has been shown to improve aerobic

Table 1
Genetic classification of OI

Gene Mutation	Protein Encoded	OI Type	Inheritance	Clinical Characteristics
COL1A1 or COL1A2	Collagen α1 or α1	I, II, III, or IV	AD	Classic phenotypes as described by Sillence classification
IFITM5	Bone-restricted IFITM-like (BRIL), also known as interferon-induced transmembrane protein 5 (IFITM5)	V	AD	Characterized by intraosseous membrane calcification and radial head dislocation
SERPINF1	Pigment epithelium-derived factor (PEDF)	VI	AR	Moderate to severe skeletal deformity
CRTAP	Cartilage-associated protein (CRTAP)	VII	AR	White sclerae; typically severe phenotype
P3H1 (also known as LEPRE1)	Prolyl-3-hydroxylase (P3H1)	VIII	AR	Severe phenotype
PPIB	Peptidyl-prolyl cis-trans isomerase B	IX	AR	Severe deformity; gray sclerae
SERPINH1	Serpin H1	X	AR	Severe skeletal deformity; gray sclerae; dentinogenesis imperfecta
FKBP10	FKBP65	XI	AR	Bruck syndrome
PLOD2	Lysyl hydroxylase 2 (LH2)	N/A	AR	Bruck syndrome
BMP1	Bone morphogenic protein 1	XII	AR	Mild to moderate skeletal deformity
SP7	Transcription factor SP7 (osterix)	XIII	AR	Severe deformity; facial hypoplasia
TMEM38B	Trimeric intracellular cation channel type B (TRIC-B)	XIV	AR	Severe bone deformity
WNT1	Proto-oncogene Wnt-1	XV	AR, AD	Severe deformity; white sclerae
CREB3L1	OASIS	XVI	AR	Severe bone deformity
SPARC	SPARC (osteonectin)	XVII	AR	Progressive severe bone fragility
MBTPS2	Membrane-bound transcription factor site-2 protease	XVIII	X-linked recessive	Moderate to severe skeletal deformity, scoliosis, pectoral deformity

Abbreviations: AD, autosomal dominant; AR, autosomal recessive.
Adapted from Marini JC, Forlino A, Bächinger HP, et al. Osteogenesis imperfecta. Nat Rev Dis Primers 2017;3:17052; with permission.

capacity and muscle force.[16–18] Furthermore, the importance of keeping the muscles as strong as possible is highlighted by developing research showing the relationship between muscle strength and bone strength.[19]

Physical Therapy

Physical therapy plays a critical role in the care of patients with OI to maximize function. The therapy plan must be individualized according to disease severity. The goals of therapy are age and developmentally individualized.[12] For families with a new baby with OI, assistance with positioning, handling, and transportation promotes safe interaction with the baby, which is important for development and bonding. The role of frequent head turns, prone positioning when possible, and play to encourage cognitive development are to be stressed. As children continue to grow and enter school age, the goal is for them to meet developmental milestones as closely as possible to other children. Participation in activities is important for social development. We have adopted an adage, "fractures heal but lack of development does not," which expresses an important principle. For adolescents and young adults navigating larger schools and perhaps a sizable campus, maximizing mobility is important and may include the use of ambulatory aids. The focus is independence and the therapist plays an important role in logistical ways to enhance independent living and the performance of activities of daily living.

Physical therapy can address common gait deviations in OI, which include increased external hip rotation, decreased strength of the hip flexors and abductors, and decreased push-off strength.[20] Exercises for core and hip girdle strengthening may be emphasized as part of a routine home exercise program.

Orthotics

The role of orthotics and braces must be considered on a case-by-case basis and reassessed regularly. For the lower extremity, ankle foot orthoses may play a role in the prevention of equinus contractures. Longer braces, such as hip-knee-ankle foot orthoses, are rarely used. Pes planovalgus of varying degrees of severity is common in patients with OI. Not all patients with pes planovalgus require orthotics and orthotics do not change the shape of the foot; however, they may be used to facilitate activity and decrease pain for some patients. There is a limited role for orthotics in the upper extremity other than as an aid to fracture management.

Fracture Management

A significant portion of fracture care for children with OI takes place in the home setting. Parents and caregivers provide the first line of evaluation and management of injuries and fractures. Home splinting provides the initial stabilization of a fracture and in doing so often controls the pain. Parents must be instructed in appropriate home splinting and pain management and a plan should be in place to seek timely orthopedic care when needed while minimizing the need for visits to the emergency room or urgent care setting. Most fracture management is nonoperative with appropriate splinting or casting. Patients should be mobilized as early as possible to minimize disuse osteopenia and loss of muscle strength and minimize the risk of refracture. Prolonged immobilization may lead to disuse osteopenia causing weakening of the bones, predisposing to another fracture. Resumption of activity as soon as possible is encouraged and may include aquatic and land-based therapies as able and progressed as tolerated.

Operative Management of Extremities

Surgical intervention plays a role in the management of progressive long bone deformity that is interfering with motor development or function or associated with recurrent fractures. A focus on developmental and functional considerations is to be emphasized over a particular age criterion for realignment and rodding of a long bone segment (**Fig. 1**). It is certainly preferable to medically optimize the bone quality preoperatively when possible. For the ambulatory patient, a gait analysis may play an important role in preoperative planning. Attention to soft tissue contractures must also be taken into consideration in surgical planning.

The technical goals of surgery are stability and alignment of an extremity. Sofield[21] pioneered the concept of multiple osteotomies and intramedullary fixation to realign and stabilize the long bones of children with OI. This surgical concept continues to be used widely, albeit with less invasive osteotomy techniques guided by intraoperative fluoroscopy.[22] The mainstay of surgical fixation of the pathologic bones of patients with OI has been intramedullary in nature, avoiding the stress risers created by a stand-alone plate and screw construct.[23] Fixed-length rods have been described, and several telescopic rods, such as the Bailey-Dubow, Sheffield, and Fassier-Duval rods.[24–28] The poor bone quality in the setting of OI renders surgical fixation challenging. A recent meta-analysis of

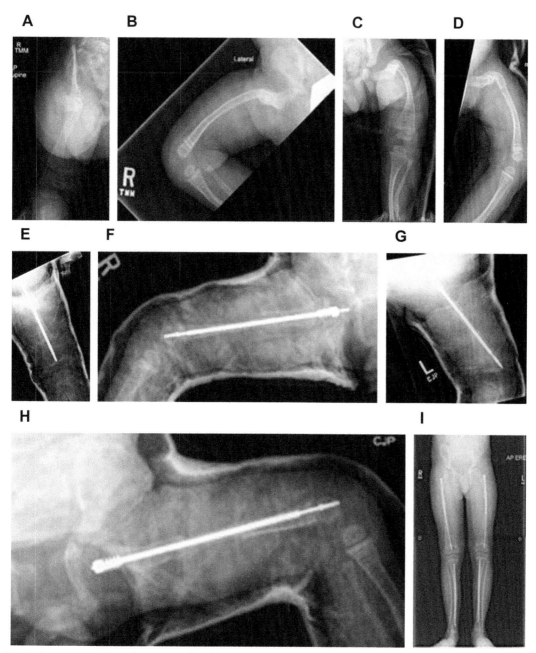

Fig. 1. Lower extremity realignment and rodding. (*A, C*) Anteroposterior (AP) and (*B, D*) lateral radiographs of the femurs of a 16-month-old boy with OI and severe femoral deformity interfering with motor development. (*E–H*) Postoperative AP and lateral radiographs following realignment and intramedullary rodding of the bilateral femurs. (*I*) Standing AP view of the lower extremities at 7 years of age demonstrates the telescopic expansion of the bilateral femoral Fassier-Duval rods with growth and interval nontelescopic realignment and intramedullary rodding of the bilateral tibias.

359 primary nonelongating rodding procedures of femurs and tibiae in children with OI with a mean follow-up of 63 months (24–118 months) found a reoperation rate of 39.4%.[29] Rod migration was the most common complication with a rate of 25.7%. The aim of telescopic rods, such as the Fassier-Duval rod, is to reduce the number of revisions required because of growth. Telescopic rods are, however, also notable for a similar revision and complication rate.[27] In their recent report on follow-up of mid-term results of femoral and tibial osteotomies and Fassier-Duval

nailing in children with OI, Azzam and colleagues[30] reported on 58 patients with 179 Fassier-Duval rods placed with a revision rate of 53% at a mean time of 52 months after initial rodding surgery. The bending of Fassier-Duval rods, not always at the male-female junction, has been described.[31] Another surgical difficulty is stress shielding.[32] Too large a rod causes stress shielding of the long bone, whereas too small a rod may bend and break (Fig. 2). Choosing intramedullary rod size is therefore somewhat controversial.

Nonunion and delayed union, particularly in the tibia, are challenges in the OI population.[30,33] The use of supplemental plate and screw fixation has been described to enhance rotational stability and serve as a tool to treat nonunions.[34–36] Some authors recommend routine removal of supplemental plates.[35] The long-term fate of these supplemental plates and screws is yet to be reported. Supplemental allogenic bone grafting may be used as an adjunct to fixation in the setting of nonunion repairs or revisions notable for bone loss.[37,38]

In patients with malalignment of the lower extremities without significant bowing of the long bones, guided growth techniques may serve a role to improve alignment during the growing years. As more centers are using these strategies, data on the effectiveness and complication rates will likely be soon to follow.

Upper extremity surgery in OI is performed to address functional limitations and has been shown to lead to functional improvements. In two recent series, Ashby and colleagues[39,40] recently reported on the functional improvements in their patients with OI who have undergone humeral and forearm rodding. Particularly in a population often reliant on wheelchairs for mobility and upper extremity function for activities of daily living, transfers, and self-care, the role of upper extremity function is important. Furthermore, as the importance of activity is emphasized for patients with OI of all severities,

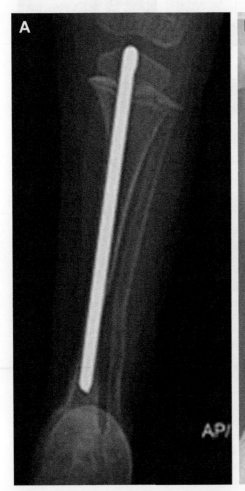
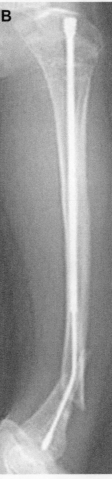

Fig. 2. Rod size: bending and breaking versus stress shielding. (A) 2-year-old ambulatory girl with a 4-mm Rush rod in the left tibia with diaphyseal stress shielding. (B) A 13-year-old ambulatory boy outgrew a 4.0-mm Fassier-Duval rod placed 5 years prior.

wheelchair sports highlight the importance of upper extremity function. Grossman and colleagues[41] report a single-center experience treating humeral deformity and fractures in children with OI using the Fassier-Duval system with a mean follow-up time of 43 months with approximately one-third requiring revision. Humeral rodding has been described with antegrade and retrograde techniques.[41,42]

Additional Extremity Considerations

In addition to deformity of the long bone segments, patients with severe OI may develop deformity of the joints. Acetabular protrusio, protrusion of the femoral head into the pelvis with envelopment of the femoral head by the acetabulum, has been described and associated with coxa vara and femoral neck fractures (**Fig. 3**).[43–45] Impingement of the acetabulum on the femoral neck may also cause hip pain with abduction. Preventative measures and effective surgical interventions for this often-dramatic phenomenon are unfortunately lacking at this time. The presence of acetabular protrusio must also be considered in the adult patient with OI with symptomatic degenerative joint disease of the hip considering arthroplasty. A similar finding takes place in the shoulder such that the humeral head becomes enveloped within the overlying acromion process with an associated deformity of the distal third of the clavicle and may be considered as shoulder protrusio (see **Fig. 3**). The effect of this phenomenon on shoulder range of motion or potential

rotator cuff or other pathology is not yet known and under investigation. In the elbow, radial head dislocation and subluxation is commonly noted and is more common in OI type V.[46] Dislocation of the radial head may be related to bowing in the forearm, although not all patients with severe forearm deformity develop a radial head dislocation (**Fig. 4**).

SPINAL DEFORMITY IN OSTEOGENESIS IMPERFECTA

Spinal manifestations include scoliosis; kyphosis; craniocervical junction (CVJ) abnormalities, such as basilar impression, basilar invagination, and platybasia; and lumbosacral pathology, such as spondylolisthesis.[47] Bisphosphonate therapy has been found to have a positive impact on vertebral morphology, including remodeling of deformed vertebrae in older children and preservation of vertebral shape when started early in life.[48,49]

Scoliosis

The prevalence of scoliosis in patients with OI ranges from 39% to 80%, depending on the study.[47] Scoliosis is rarely observed in patients younger than 6 years and can progress rapidly after it is diagnosed.[50] Single thoracic curves are the most frequent type of scoliosis curve found in patients with type I OI: 97% of curves in patients with type I OI who have scoliosis are single thoracic curves, whereas in patients with type III OI, 58% of curves are in the thoracic region.[51]

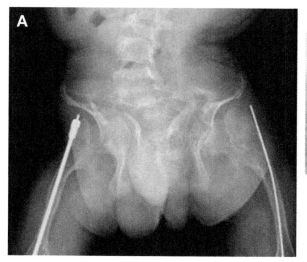 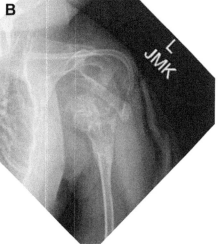

Fig. 3. Acetabular and shoulder protrusio. (*A*) A 12-year-old boy with severe OI with bilateral acetabular protrusio. (*B*) A 17-year-old boy with severe OI with left shoulder protrusion characterized by envelopment of the humeral head in the acromion process.

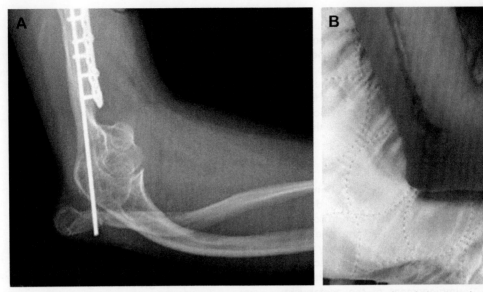

Fig. 4. Radial head dislocation. (*A*) Lateral radiograph of the right elbow and (*B*) a clinical photograph of the right elbow of a 17-year-old boy with a right radial head dislocation.

The cause of scoliosis in patients with OI is controversial, with theories including vertebral body fragility, vertebral body shape, ligamentous laxity, muscle weakness, limb-length discrepancy, and pelvic obliquity.[52,53] Vertebral fractures are thought to be a leading cause of scoliosis because of the severe fragility of the vertebral growth plates and the progression that occurs with continued growth.[54] Benson and Newman[50] and Engelbert and colleagues[55] theorized that ligamentous laxity plays a substantial role because the lack of stability between vertebrae allows scoliosis to progress.

Untreated scoliosis is known to progress in growing children with OI and even into adulthood.[53] Scoliosis curve progression is 6° per year in patients with type III OI, 4° per year in patients with type IV OI, and 1° per year in patients with type I OI.[51] Watanabe and colleagues[52] found that, as the DEXA *z* score worsened, the scoliosis progressed, suggesting that poorer bone quality leads to more severe scoliosis. Ishikawa and colleagues[54] found that biconcave vertebrae, in which the height of the midportion of the body is less than 70% of the mean of the anterior and posterior vertebral body heights, were common in patients with OI (**Fig. 5**). The presence of six or more biconcave vertebrae before puberty suggested that severe scoliosis would develop.

Anissipour and colleagues[51] found that patients with type III OI who began bisphosphonate treatment before age 6 years had slower curve progression after the development of scoliosis than did patients who started

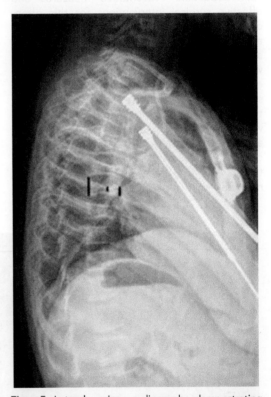

Fig. 5. Lateral spine radiograph demonstrating osteogenesis imperfecta in a 5-year-old boy. The patient has multiple biconcave vertebrae. For T7, the anterior vertebral body height is 11 mm, the posterior vertebral body height is 6.9 mm, and the midportion vertebral body height is 4.6 mm. Black lines indicate vertebral body height measurement locations. The height of the midportion of the body is 51% of the mean of the anterior and posterior vertebral body heights.

bisphosphonate treatment after age 6 years (2.3° per year vs 6° per year). Bisphosphonate treatment started after age 6 years or in patients with type I or IV OI did not have a statistically significant effect on the progression of scoliosis.

Widmann and colleagues[47] evaluated patients with OI and found that increasing severity of scoliosis correlated with a decrease in pulmonary function, specifically the vital capacity, leading to restrictive lung disease. Vital capacity was 78% predicted when thoracic scoliosis was less than 40° and dropped to 41% predicted when thoracic scoliosis was greater than 60°. The authors did not find a correlation between pulmonary function and kyphosis or chest wall deformity.

Treatment of scoliosis in patients with OI is difficult mostly because of poor bone quality and the rigidity of the deformity. Brace treatment has not been found to be effective and is difficult to use because of the fragility of the rib cage. In some patients, a soft thoracolumbosacral orthosis is used for supported sitting to assist with functional activities, but no assurance should be given with regard to curve progression.

Surgical spinal fusion to halt curve progression is considered when curves reach 45°, but the patient's age and truncal height need to be taken into account to avoid thoracic insufficiency syndrome. One report indicated that children with severe OI may benefit from fusion when curves are 35°,[56] but it is preferable to avoid fusion in young children when possible because contemporary techniques make correction of larger curves at a later stage more feasible. Although historical methods of fusion have not been found to improve lung volumes, contemporary techniques may improve results, and fusion can prevent progressive respiratory decline resulting from thoracic insufficiency syndrome.[47]

Previous methods of treatment, including noninstrumented fusion, Harrington rods, and Luque instrumentation, have shown modest or no correction of curves, little improvement in physical function, and up to 50% complication rates.[50,53,55,57–59] Recent evaluation of contemporary instrumentation and correction techniques, such as the use of pedicle screws with cement augmentation, has shown improved outcomes. Yilmaz and colleagues[60] reviewed a series of 10 patients with OI who underwent posterior spinal fusion for the treatment of scoliosis. All of the patients underwent preoperative pamidronate therapy. Seven patients had cement-augmented pedicle screw instrumentation at the proximal and distal foundations (Fig. 6). These authors were the first to report the difficulty of exposure of the thoracic spine because of rib overgrowth and thoracic lordosis (Fig. 7). Rib and posterior Ponte osteotomies at the apex of the thoracic curve were used to aid in adequate exposure and to increase flexibility of the curve in the coronal and sagittal planes to allow correction. Cement augmentation of the proximal and distal screws was used to increase pullout strength of fixation

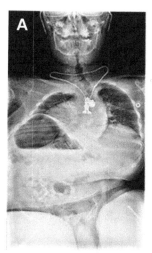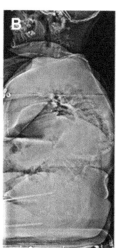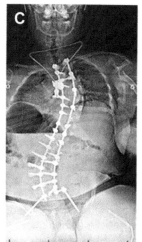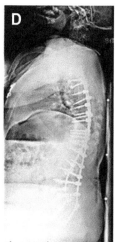

Fig. 6. (A) Posteroanterior (PA) and (B) lateral radiographs demonstrating severe osteogenesis imperfecta in a 16-year-old boy with an 87° thoracic curve, a 115° thoracolumbar curve, and substantial pelvic obliquity. (C) PA and (D) lateral radiographs obtained 2.5 years postoperatively demonstrate spinal fusion from T1 to the sacrum with cement-augmented pedicle screws and pelvic fixation.

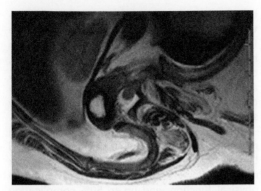

Fig. 7. Preoperative T2-weighted axial MRI demonstrating type III osteogenesis imperfecta in a 19-year-old man. Note the severe rib deformities that made access to the posterior spinal elements challenging. Multiple rib osteotomies were required during posterior spinal fusion to gain adequate access to the posterior elements for pedicle screw placement and Ponte osteotomies to aid in correction of the deformity.

in bone. An average correction of 48% was reported with no loss of correction at follow-up, no neurologic deficits, and no implant failures. Improved quality of life scores, pain, and sitting tolerance were also noted.[60]

Authors' preferred treatment strategy

Children with OI are followed at least annually for clinical signs of spinal deformity. For those with curves greater than 30°, more frequent follow-up is recommended, especially during peak height velocity. Current indications for fusion are curves greater than 50° in patients who are past peak height velocity or patients with substantial curve progression after skeletal maturity because these curves can continue to progress in adulthood. Curve rigidity is an important factor in the timing of surgical treatment and is evaluated clinically. We observe curves that progress during growth if they remain flexible. The proximal extent of instrumentation and fusion is usually T2, T3, or T4 and depends on the stable vertebra in the coronal plane and the extent of proximal thoracic kyphosis. The distal extent of fusion is the vertebra that is stable on the erect radiograph, unless the sagittal plane demonstrates an indication for lower fusion, such as thoracolumbar junctional kyphosis. In addition to apical lordosis, compensatory kyphosis above and below the apex of the thoracic and thoracolumbar curves is problematic and needs to be addressed in the selection of fusion levels. Proximal instrumentation and fusion to T2, T3, or T4 is frequently needed to control the sagittal plane and prevent proximal junctional kyphosis. Pelvic fixation is sometimes indicated for the management of severe pelvic obliquity.

In patients with rigid, severe (90°) curves, preoperative traction is occasionally used to avoid the need for three-column osteotomy and to achieve slow correction over time. Intraoperative traction may help achieve slow correction with release of the facets and intersegmental ligaments (interspinous, ligamentum flavum) and viscoelastic creep and to address the deformity in all three planes. Traction may decrease the force that the instrumentation needs to exert on the spinal column. Exposure of the spine in patients with severe rib deformity, especially those with thoracic lordosis, sometimes requires rib osteotomy and retraction. All patients are monitored intraoperatively with multimodal spinal cord monitoring consisting of transcranial motor-evoked potentials, somatosensory-evoked potentials, and electromyography.

In our opinion, pamidronate therapy results in more robust cortical bone in the spine and improves pullout strength of pedicle screw fixation when screws appropriately fill the pedicle. Pamidronate therapy does not seem to affect the intraoperative appearance of the bone or the risk of bleeding. Because bisphosphonates affect bone remodeling, continuation of pamidronate therapy can theoretically affect the quality of the fusion. However, no evidence-based guidelines in the literature address the perioperative use of bisphosphonates. We prefer to withhold pamidronate for 4 months postoperatively to facilitate partial resumption of osteoclast function to allow for remodeling of the fusion mass. If postoperative surveillance radiographs indicate early signs of fusion and the implants are stable, pamidronate therapy is resumed.

Craniocervical Junction Abnormalities

CVJ abnormalities are observed in 37% of patients with OI; these abnormalities include basilar invagination, basilar impression, and platybasia (seen in 13%, 15%, and 29% of patients with OI, respectively) and secondary hydrocephalus.[61] Basilar invagination is protrusion of the uppermost cervical structures into the foramen magnum with projection of the tip of the dens greater than 5 mm above the Chamberlain line (from the posterior nasal spine to the posterior lip of the foramen magnum) or greater than 7 mm above the McGregor line (from the posterior nasal spine to the most caudal portion of the posterior cranial base). Basilar impression is relative lowering of the cranial base (occipital condyles and foramen magnum) with resultant positioning of the uppermost cervical vertebral

structures above the caudal border of the skull. Platybasia is flattening of the cranial base.[61,62] A recent study demonstrated skull base abnormalities in all four types of OI with 26% of patients having at least one abnormality; 16% had platybasia, 6% had basilar impression, and 4% had basilar invagination. Increased clinical severity of OI was the strongest predictor of skull base anomalies. This retrospective review demonstrated that treatment within the first year of life with bisphosphonates did not decrease the prevalence of skull base abnormalities later in life.[63]

Basilar impression results in characteristic features of the skull. These features include overhang of the temporal and occipital bones, termed the "Tam-o'-Shanter" or "Darth Vader" skull.[64] Clinical presentation of CVJ problems can range from no symptoms to brainstem compression, restriction of cerebrospinal fluid circulation resulting in hydrocephalus, and impingement of cranial nerves.[65] Baseline lateral skull/cervical spine radiographs are recommended in all patients with OI before they reach age 6 years. Basilar impression may be clearly visible on a lateral radiograph with upward migration of the cervical spine into the base of the skull. In more subtle cases, the diagnosis of basilar invagination is made when the odontoid process protrudes above the Chamberlain, McRae, and McGregor lines on the lateral radiograph (Figs. 8A, B).[64] Drawing the recommended lines on plain radiographs is challenging because of the deformity and overlapping bony detail. If craniocervical abnormalities are a substantial concern, MRI is recommended (Fig. 8C).

Treatment of symptomatic CVJ problems includes craniocervical fusion with or without traction (Fig. 9). Sawin and Menezes[66] reported on 25 patients with basilar invagination, 18 of whom had OI. Of the 25 patients, 56% were between ages 11 and 15 years, and 44% also had symptoms of hydrocephalus. Patients with asymptomatic basilar invagination were treated with external orthotic immobilization. Symptomatic patients with hydrocephalus underwent ventriculoperitoneal shunt placement before treatment of basilar invagination. The treatment of the CVJ abnormality depended on whether the basilar invagination was successfully reduced with preoperative traction. The patients in whom reduction occurred (40%) were treated with posterior decompression and occipitocervical fusion with or without instrumentation. The patients in whom reduction did not occur (60%) underwent transoral or transnasal anterior decompression,

followed by posterior occipitocervical fusion. These patients were treated with in situ occipitocervical fusion with autogenous rib strut grafting with sublaminar cables or contoured loop instrumentation. Postoperatively, all patients used either a halo vest or modified Minerva braces until solid union was observed. Contemporary rigid occipitocervical instrumentation was not used in this series. Although successful fusion occurred at an average of 8.2 months postoperatively, progression of the basilar invagination was observed in 80% of the patients. Of the 20 patients with progression, six patients were symptomatic; these patients were treated with prolonged external bracing with improvement over time.

Authors' preferred treatment strategy
Our indication for surgical treatment abnormalities is generally reserved for invagination with clinical symptoms commonly including headaches, cranial palsy, dysphagia, and myelopathy hyperreflexia, quadriparesis, or gait Hydrocephalus in patients with basilar invagination is dangerous and must be t any other intervention is performed history of basilar invagination c gressive deformity and neurolog creating the controversy of whe treatment is indicated in asym with basilar invagination evi We take a conservative sta monitor patients who are development of neurolog can be subtle and can pr not think that the literatu evidence that the use of a progression of basilar i symptomatic basilar inv No definitive eviden proven that delayed s basilar invagination upright posture is n tients with OI beca are motivated to s near normal deve

Lumbosacral P
Spondylolysis found in patie the L5 level. In from 5.3% to evaluated la with OI to spondyloly 8.2% inci age of 7

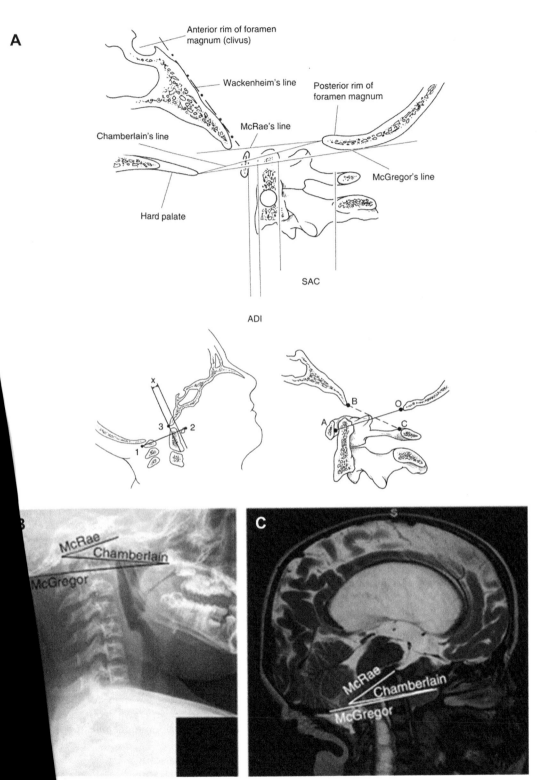

Diagram depicting the Chamberlain line, which extends from the posterior nasal spine to the posterior [fo]ramen magnum; the McRae line, which joins the anterior and posterior margins of the foramen mag[num, th]e McGregor line, which extends from the posterior nasal spine to the most caudal portion of the pos[terior] base. (B) Lateral cervical spine radiograph demonstrating type III osteogenesis imperfecta in a [g]irl. This image demonstrates the difficulty of drawing the McGregor, Chamberlain, and McRae lines. [McRae li]ne was difficult to draw because the anterior and posterior aspects of the foramen magnum were [difficult to vis]ualize. (C) Sagittal T2-weighted MRI was obtained for further evaluation of the same patient. The [McRae, Ch]amberlain, and McRae lines are drawn. Hydrocephalus and syrinx are present. ADI, atlantodens in-[terval; SAC, sp]ace available for spinal cord. ([A] From Wills BP, Dormans JP. Nontraumatic upper cervical spine [injuries in ch]ildren. J Am Acad Orthop Surg 2006;14(4):237; with permission.)

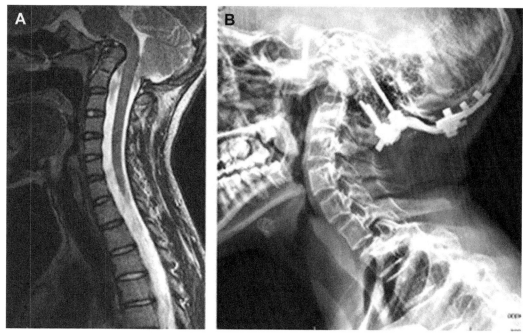

Fig. 9. (*A*) T2-weighted sagittal MRI demonstrating progressive basilar invagination in a 14-year-old boy with osteogenesis imperfecta. The patient had headaches, neck pain, and decreased endurance but no overt symptoms of myelopathy. (*B*) Postoperative lateral radiograph of the same patient demonstrates occiput to C2 fusion, which was performed with intraoperative traction.

ambulatory. Spondylolisthesis occurred in 12 patients (10.9%) at an average age of 6.4 years, with 92% of those patients ambulatory. Eleven of these 12 instances of spondylolisthesis occurred at L5/S1, and one was at S1/S2. Nine were isthmic spondylolisthesis, and three were dysplastic. The grade was low in 10 patients and high in two patients. The authors did not find that one specific type of OI had a higher incidence of spondylolisthesis than other types, although seven of the nine patients with spondylolysis had type III OI.

The clinical relevance and natural history of spondylolysis and spondylolisthesis in patients with OI are not clear in the literature, and information on surgical indications and techniques is available only in sparse case reports. In our experience, many patients with OI do not have normal pelvic parameters and often have increased lumbar lordosis, and an increase in lumbar lordosis can even develop at the distal end of a fusion construct (**Figs. 10** and **11**). The practitioner also needs to be aware of hip flexion contractures and the possibility of acetabular protrusio.

ANESTHETIC AND INTRAOPERATIVE CONSIDERATIONS

The surgeon must be aware of several anesthetic and intraoperative considerations in patients with OI. Fractures can occur when patients are transferred to the surgical table, positioned, during the procedure, and transferred to the postoperative bed. In severely affected

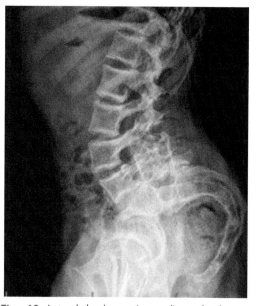

Fig. 10. Lateral lumbar spine radiograph demonstrating osteogenesis imperfecta in a 20-year-old woman who reported increasing low back pain. The patient has substantial lumbar lordosis, elongated pedicles, and a horizontal sacrum with sacral deformity.

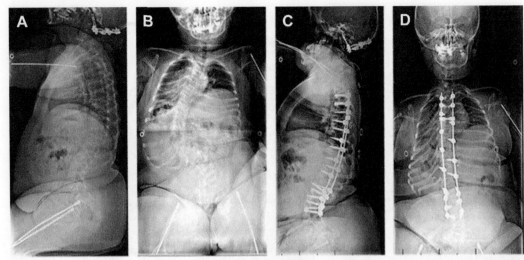

Fig. 11. (A) Lateral and (B) PA radiographs demonstrating increased lumbar lordosis in a 16-year-old girl with osteogenesis imperfecta and scoliosis. (C) Postoperative lateral and (D) PA radiographs obtained 2 years after fusion demonstrate distal lordosis at the end of the fusion construct.

patients, fractures can result from the use of blood pressure cuffs and from tourniquets used for insertion of intravenous lines. Airway management in anesthesia is challenging because these patients often have large heads, large tongues, and short necks. They also have poor pulmonary function as a result of chest wall deformities. Normal lung predictions based on age and size are not accurate in patients with OI because of their stature. Hyperthermia and diaphoresis tend to occur in these patients. The use of succinylcholine should be avoided because fasciculations can cause fractures in severely affected patients.[64] Patients with OI can lose substantial amounts of blood during spinal surgery; therefore, blood should be available for transfusion if required. Controlled hypotension during the spinal exposure and use of tranexamic acid can decrease blood loss and have been shown to be effective in the surgical management of complex pediatric spinal deformity.[69]

REFERENCES

1. Morello R. Osteogenesis imperfecta and therapeutics. Matrix Biol 2018;71-72:294–312.
2. Marini JC, Forlino A, Bächinger HP, et al. Osteogenesis imperfecta. Nat Rev Dis Primers 2017. https://doi.org/10.1038/nrdp.2017.52.
3. Vrolik W. Tabulae Ad Illustrandam Embryogenesin Hominis et Mammalium Tam Naturalem Tam Abnormem; 1849.
4. Baljet B. Aspects of the history of osteogenesis imperfecta (Vrolik's syndrome). Ann Anat 2002. https://doi.org/10.1016/S0940-9602(02)80023-1.
5. Sillence DO, Senn A, Danks DM. Genetic heterogeneity in osteogenesis imperfecta. J Med Genet 1979. https://doi.org/10.1136/jmg.16.2.101.
6. Barsh GS, Byers PH. Reduced secretion of structurally abnormal type I procollagen in a form of osteogenesis imperfecta. Proc Natl Acad Sci U S A 1981. https://doi.org/10.1073/pnas.78.8.5142.
7. Chu ML, Williams CJ, Pepe G, et al. Internal deletion in a collagen gene in a perinatal lethal form of osteogenesis imperfecta. Nature 1983. https://doi.org/10.1038/304078a0.
8. Barnes AM, Chang W, Morello R, et al. Deficiency of cartilage-associated protein in recessive lethal osteogenesis imperfecta. N Engl J Med 2006. https://doi.org/10.1056/NEJMoa063804.
9. Glorieux FH, Rauch F, Plotkin H, et al. Type V osteogenesis imperfecta: a new form of brittle bone disease. J Bone Miner Res 2000. https://doi.org/10.1359/jbmr.2000.15.9.1650.
10. Van Dijk FS, Sillence DO. Osteogenesis imperfecta: clinical diagnosis, nomenclature and severity assessment. Am J Med Genet A 2014. https://doi.org/10.1002/ajmg.a.36545.
11. Smith PA, Rauch FHG, editors. Transitional care in osteogenesis imperfecta: advances in biology, technology, and clinical practice. Chicago (IL): Shriners Hospitals for Children - Chicago; 2015.
12. Marr C, Seasman A, Bishop N. Managing the patient with osteogenesis imperfecta: a multidisciplinary approach. J Multidiscip Healthc 2017. https://doi.org/10.2147/JMDH.S113483.
13. Sakkers R, Kok D, Engelbert R, et al. Skeletal effects and functional outcome with olpadronate in children with osteogenesis imperfecta: a 2-year randomised placebo-controlled study. Lancet 2004. https://doi.org/10.1016/S0140-6736(04)16101-1.

14. Dwan K, Phillipi CA, Steiner RD, et al. Bisphosphonate therapy for osteogenesis imperfecta. Cochrane Database Syst Rev 2016. https://doi.org/10.1002/14651858.CD005088.pub4.

15. Olvera D, Stolzenfeld R, Marini JC, et al. Low dose of bisphosphonate enhances sclerostin antibody-induced trabecular bone mass gains in Brtl/+ osteogenesis imperfecta mouse model. J Bone Miner Res 2018. https://doi.org/10.1002/jbmr.3421.

16. Engelbert RH, Uiterwaal CS, Gerver WJ, et al. Osteogenesis imperfecta in childhood: impairment and disability. a prospective study with 4-year follow-up. Arch Phys Med Rehabil 2004. https://doi.org/10.1016/j.apmr.2003.08.085.

17. Van Brussel M, Takken T, Uiterwaal CSPM, et al. Physical training in children with osteogenesis imperfecta. J Pediatr 2008. https://doi.org/10.1016/j.jpeds.2007.06.029.

18. Veilleux LN, Lemay M, Pouliot-Laforte A, et al. Muscle anatomy and dynamic muscle function in osteogenesis imperfecta type I. J Clin Endocrinol Metab 2014. https://doi.org/10.1210/jc.2013-3209.

19. Veilleux LN, Pouliot-Laforte A, Lemay M, et al. The functional muscle-bone unit in patients with osteogenesis imperfecta type I. Bone 2015. https://doi.org/10.1016/j.bone.2015.05.019.

20. Garman CR, Graf A, Krzak J, et al. Gait deviations in children with osteogenesis imperfecta type I. J Pediatr Orthop 2017. https://doi.org/10.1097/BPO.0000000000001062.

21. Sofield HA ME. Fragmentation, realignment, and intramedullary rod fixation of deformities of the long bones in children: a ten year appraisal. J Bone Joint Surg Am 1959;41-A(8):1371–91.

22. Esposito P, Plotkin H. Surgical treatment of osteogenesis imperfecta: current concepts. Curr Opin Pediatr 2008. https://doi.org/10.1097/MOP.0b013e3282f35f03.

23. Enright WJ, Noonan KJ. Bone plating in patients with type III osteogenesis imperfecta: results and complications. Iowa Orthop J 2006;26:37–40.

24. Karbowski A, Schwitalle M, Brenner R, et al. Experience with Bailey-Dubow rodding in children with osteogenesis imperfecta. Eur J Pediatr Surg 2000. https://doi.org/10.1055/s-2008-1072339.

25. Stockley I, Bell MJ, Sharrard WJW. The role of expanding intramedullary rods in osteogenesis imperfecta. J Bone Joint Surg Br 1989. https://doi.org/10.1016/S0022-3468(05)80238-6.

26. Marafioti RL, Westin GW. Elongating intramedullary rods in the treatment of osteogenesis imperfecta. J Bone Joint Surg Am 1977. https://doi.org/10.2106/00004623-197759040-00006.

27. Birke O, Davies N, Latimer M, et al. Experience with the Fassier-Duval telescopic rod: first 24 consecutive cases with a minimum of 1-year follow-up. J Pediatr Orthop 2011. https://doi.org/10.1097/BPO.0b013e31821bfb50.

28. Nicolaou N, Bowe JD, Wilkinson JM, et al. Use of the Sheffield telescopic intramedullary rod system for the management of osteogenesis imperfecta: clinical outcomes at an average follow-up of nineteen years. J Bone Joint Surg Am 2011. https://doi.org/10.2106/JBJS.J.01893.

29. Scollan JP, Jauregui JJ, Jacobsen CM, et al. The outcomes of nonelongating intramedullary fixation of the lower extremity for pediatric osteogenesis imperfecta patients: a meta-analysis. J Pediatr Orthop 2017. https://doi.org/10.1097/BPO.0000000000000970.

30. Azzam KA, Rush ET, Burke BR, et al. Mid-term results of femoral and tibial osteotomies and fassier-duval nailing in children with osteogenesis imperfecta. J Pediatr Orthop 2018. https://doi.org/10.1097/BPO.0000000000000824.

31. Lee RJ, Paloski MD, Sponseller PD, et al. Bent telescopic rods in patients with osteogenesis imperfecta. J Pediatr Orthop 2016. https://doi.org/10.1097/BPO.0000000000000509.

32. Reing CM. Report on new types of intramedullary rods and treatment effectiveness data for selection of intramedullary rodding in osteogenesis imperfecta. Connect Tissue Res 1995. https://doi.org/10.3109/03008209509116839.

33. Agarwal V, Joseph B. Non-union in osteogenesis imperfecta. J Pediatr Orthop B 2005. https://doi.org/10.1097/01202412-200511000-00013.

34. Hsiao CMS, Mormino MA, Esposito PW, et al. Distal humerus atrophic nonunion in a child with osteogenesis imperfecta. J Pediatr Orthop 2013. https://doi.org/10.1097/BPO.0b013e3182a32e69.

35. Cho TJ, Lee K, Oh CW, et al. Locking plate placement with unicortical screw fixation adjunctive to intramedullary rodding in long bones of patients with osteogenesis imperfecta. J Bone Joint Surg Am 2015. https://doi.org/10.2106/JBJS.N.01185.

36. Franzone JM, Kruse RW. Intramedullary nailing with supplemental plate and screw fixation of long bones of patients with osteogenesis imperfecta: operative technique and preliminary results. J Pediatr Orthop B 2018. https://doi.org/10.1097/BPB.0000000000000405.

37. Puvanesarajah V, Shapiro JR, Sponseller PD, et al. Sandwich allografts for long-bone nonunions in patients with osteogenesis imperfecta: a retrospective study. J Bone Joint Surg Am 2015. https://doi.org/10.2106/JBJS.N.00584.

38. Vlad C, Georgescu I, Gavriliu TS, et al. Burnei's procedure in the treatment of long bone pseudarthrosis in patients having osteogenesis imperfecta or congenital pseudarthrosis of tibia: preliminary report. J Med Life 2012;5(2):215–21.

39. Ashby E, Montpetit K, Hamdy RC, et al. Functional outcome of humeral rodding in children with osteogenesis imperfecta. J Pediatr Orthop 2018. https://doi.org/10.1097/BPO.0000000000000729.

40. Ashby E, Montpetit K, Hamdy RC, et al. Functional outcome of forearm rodding in children with osteogenesis imperfecta. J Pediatr Orthop 2018. https://doi.org/10.1097/BPO.0000000000000724.

41. Grossman LS, Price AL, Rush ET, et al. Initial experience with percutaneous IM rodding of the humeri in children with osteogenesis imperfecta. J Pediatr Orthop 2016;38(9):484–9d.

42. Franzone JM, Bober MB, Rogers KJ, et al. Re-alignment and intramedullary rodding of the humerus and forearm in children with osteogenesis imperfecta: revision rate and effect on fracture rate. J Child Orthop 2017;11(3):185–90.

43. King JDBW. Osteogenesis imperfecta: an orthopaedic description and surgical review. J Bone Joint Surg Br 1971;53(B):72–89.

44. Trehan SK, Morakis E, Raggio CL, et al. Acetabular protrusio and proximal femur fractures in patients with osteogenesis imperfecta. J Pediatr Orthop 2015;35(6):645–9.

45. Ahn J, Carter E, Raggio CL, et al. Acetabular protrusio in patients with osteogenesis imperfecta: risk factors and progression. J Pediatr Orthop 2017. https://doi.org/10.1097/BPO.0000000000001051.

46. Fassier AM, Rauch F, Aarabi M, et al. Radial head dislocation and subluxation in osteogenesis imperfecta. J Bone Joint Surg Am 2007. https://doi.org/10.2106/JBJS.F.01287.

47. Widmann RF, Bitan FD, Laplaza FJ, et al. Spinal deformity, pulmonary compromise, and quality of life in osteogenesis imperfecta. Spine (Phila Pa 1976) 1999. https://doi.org/10.1097/00007632-199908150-00008.

48. Land C, Rauch F, Munns CF, et al. Vertebral morphometry in children and adolescents with osteogenesis imperfecta: effect of intravenous pamidronate treatment. Bone 2006. https://doi.org/10.1016/j.bone.2006.04.004.

49. Semler O, Beccard R, Palmisano D, et al. Reshaping of vertebrae during treatment with neridronate or pamidronate in children with osteogenesis imperfecta. Horm Res Paediatr 2011. https://doi.org/10.1159/000331128.

50. Benson DR, Newman DC. The spine and surgical treatment in osteogenesis imperfecta. Clin Orthop Relat Res 1981;(159):147–53.

51. Anissipour AK, Hammerberg KW, Caudill A, et al. Behavior of scoliosis during growth in children with osteogenesis imperfecta. J Bone Joint Surg Am 2014. https://doi.org/10.2106/JBJS.L.01596.

52. Watanabe G, Kawaguchi S, Matsuyama T, et al. Correlation of scoliotic curvature with Z-score bone mineral density and body mass index in patients with osteogenesis imperfecta. Spine (Phila Pa 1976) 2007. https://doi.org/10.1097/BRS.0b013e31811ec2d9.

53. Yong-Hing K, MacEwen GD. Scoliosis associated with osteogenesis imperfecta. J Bone Joint Surg Br 1982. https://doi.org/10.1016/S0022-3468(83)80329-7.

54. Ishikawa S, Kumar SJ, Takahashi HE, et al. Vertebral body shape as a predictor of spinal deformity in osteogenesis imperfecta. J Bone Joint Surg Am 1996;78(2):212–9.

55. Engelbert RHH, Uiterwaal CSPM, van der Hulst A, et al. Scoliosis in children with osteogenesis imperfecta: influence of severity of disease and age of reaching motor milestones. Eur Spine J 2003. https://doi.org/10.1007/s00586-002-0491-x.

56. Kocher MS, Shapiro F. Osteogenesis imperfecta. J Am Acad Orthop Surg 1998. https://doi.org/10.5435/00124635-199807000-00004.

57. Cristofaro RL, Hoek KJ, Bonnett CA, et al. Operative treatment of spine deformity in osteogenesis imperfecta. Clin Orthop Relat Res 1978. https://doi.org/10.1097/00003086-197903000-00005.

58. Hanscom DA, Winter RB, Lutter L, et al. Osteogenesis imperfecta. Radiographic classification, natural history, and treatment of spinal deformities. J Bone Joint Surg Am 1992;74(4):598–616.

59. Janus GJM, Finidori G, Engelbert RHH, et al. Operative treatment of severe scoliosis in osteogenesis imperfecta: results of 20 patients after halo traction and posterior spondylodesis with instrumentation. Eur Spine J 2000. https://doi.org/10.1007/s005860000165.

60. Yilmaz G, Hwang S, Oto M, et al. Surgical treatment of scoliosis in osteogenesis imperfecta with cement-augmented pedicle screw instrumentation. J Spinal Disord Tech 2014. https://doi.org/10.1097/BSD.0b013e3182624b76.

61. Arponen H, Mäkitie O, Haukka J, et al. Prevalence and natural course of craniocervical junction anomalies during growth in patients with osteogenesis imperfecta. J Bone Miner Res 2012. https://doi.org/10.1002/jbmr.1555.

62. Sillence DO. Craniocervical abnormalities in osteogenesis imperfecta: genetic and molecular correlation. Pediatr Radiol 1994. https://doi.org/10.1007/BF02011910.

63. Cheung MS, Arponen H, Roughley P, et al. Cranial base abnormalities in osteogenesis imperfecta: phenotypic and genotypic determinants. J Bone Miner Res 2011. https://doi.org/10.1002/jbmr.220.

64. Lubicky J. The spine in osteogenesis imperfecta. In: Weinstein SL, editor. The pediatric spine: principles and practice. 1st edition. New York: Raven Press; 1994. p. 943–58.

65. Khandanpour N, Connolly DJA, Raghavan A, et al. Craniospinal abnormalities and neurologic complications of osteogenesis imperfecta: imaging overview. Radiographics 2012. https://doi.org/10.1148/rg.327125716.

66. Sawin PD, Menezes AH. Basilar invagination in osteogenesis imperfecta and related osteochondrodysplasias: medical and surgical management. J Neurosurg 1997. https://doi.org/10.3171/jns.1997.86.6.0950.

67. Verra WC, Pruijs HJ, Beek EJ, et al. Prevalence of vertebral pars defects (spondylolysis) in a population with osteogenesis imperfecta. Spine (Phila Pa 1976) 2009. https://doi.org/10.1097/BRS.0b013e3181a39646.

68. Hatz D, Esposito PW, Schroeder B, et al. The incidence of spondylolysis and spondylolisthesis in children with osteogenesis imperfecta. J Pediatr Orthop 2011. https://doi.org/10.1097/BPO.0b013e31822889c9.

69. Dhawale AA, Shah SA, Sponseller PD, et al. Are antifibrinolytics helpful in decreasing blood loss and transfusions during spinal fusion surgery in children with cerebral palsy scoliosis? Spine (Phila Pa 1976) 2012. https://doi.org/10.1097/BRS.0b013e31823d009b.

Hand and Wrist

Wrist Fractures and Osteoporosis

John C. Wu, MD*, Carson D. Strickland, MD, James S. Chambers, MD

KEYWORDS

• Wrist fracture • Osteoporosis • Outcomes • Treatment options • Elderly patients

KEY POINTS

- Osteoporosis is a predominant factor for low-energy distal radial fractures in the elderly.
- Distal radial fractures may be the first opportunity to evaluate and treat osteoporosis to reduce the risk of future fragility fractures.
- Treatment may involve pharmacotherapy, closed reduction and splinting or casting, external fixation, or open reduction and internal fixation.
- Published evidence supports favorable functional outcomes, regardless of the presence of osteoporosis, after volar plate fixation of distal radial fragility fractures.

Although both conservative management and surgical management have been reported to be successful, current evidence and the most recent American Academy of Orthopaedic Surgeons (AAOS) clinical guidelines comparing conservative and surgical treatment of distal radial fragility fractures are inconclusive. Each treatment method has its advantages: volar locking plate fixation allows earlier mobilization than casting, with better functional outcomes; Kirschner (K)-wire fixation can minimize the risk associated with open surgery; intramedullary fixation increases fixation strength, prevents tendon irritation, and speeds return to activity; and dorsal distraction plating allows early weight-bearing across the wrist. Treatment must be individualized based on fracture pattern, patient age, activity level, and osteoporosis severity.

Fractures caused by a low-energy mechanism in patients with poor bone quality and osteoporosis (fragility fractures) are a major health concern for the elderly population, with more than 1.5 million injuries occurring each year in the United States.[1] Osteoporosis is defined as a bone mineral density (BMD) of less than 2.5 SDs of peak bone mass below a healthy gender-matched young adult. In individuals with osteoporosis, a fall from standing can result in distal radial, proximal humeral, hip, and pelvic fractures. Fragility fractures are associated with significant morbidity and mortality and can cause disability that can ultimately lead to a loss of independence. The 1-year mortality after a hip fracture is 20% in the elderly population, and only 50% of hip fracture patients return to their previous level of function.[2,3] Although isolated distal radial fractures can cause difficulty in performing activities of daily living, they do not seem associated with increased mortality.[4] One study, however, found that women from 60 years to 79 years of age who had sustained a fracture of the distal radius or proximal humerus had a relative risk of sustaining a future hip fracture of 1.9, with the highest risk within the first year after a fracture.[5] A prospective cohort study followed 113 patients for 4 years after sustaining a distal radial fracture and found that 24% experienced a subsequent fall and 19% experienced a subsequent fracture during that time.[6,7] A distal radial fracture seems a fortunate outcome in comparison to a hip fracture in a fall, and it may serve as an early indicator for future fragility fractures and morbidity.

Osteoporosis is a predominant factor for low-energy distal radial fractures in the elderly and should not be overlooked. Disruption of the

Department of Orthopaedic Surgery and Biomedical Engineering, Campbell Clinic, University of Tennessee, 1211 Union Avenue, Suite 510, Memphis, TN 38104, USA
* Corresponding author.
E-mail address: jwu@campbellclinic.com

Orthop Clin N Am 50 (2019) 211–221
https://doi.org/10.1016/j.ocl.2018.10.004
0030-5898/19/

balance between bone formation and resorption leads to an age-related decrease in bone mass and eventual osteoporosis. Decreased activity, hormonal changes, and vitamin D and calcium deficiency are factors that contribute to osteoporosis in the elderly. Patients with distal radial fractures have been found to have an increased level of bone turnover markers of formation and resorption.[1] Rozental and colleagues suggested that these turnover markers may be helpful in predicting future fragility fractures in premenopausal women. In a comparison of patients who were and were not receiving hormonal treatment, the risk of a distal radial fracture was reduced by 33% in those who had hormonal treatment for 10 years and by 63% in those who used them for 15 years.[8] The study also showed that long-term hormonal therapy protected bone loss and reduced the frequency of wrist fractures. Hormonal therapy of less than 5 years did not have a long-term protective effect, but the study was under-powered to confirm this result.

DEMOGRAPHICS OF AND RISK FACTORS FOR DISTAL RADIAL FRACTURES

Distal radial fractures account for up to 18% of all fractures in patients over 65 years of age.[9] Risk factors include female gender, obesity, frequent falls, white race, and diagnosis of osteoporosis.[10] The prevalence of osteoporosis in patients with distal radial fractures is high compared with matched control subjects, regardless of gender.[11] A study from Canada demonstrated that all participants older than 65 years of age were at moderate or high risk for an osteoporotic fracture when using the fracture risk assessment and Canadian Association of Radiologists–Osteoporosis Canada risk assessment tools.[12] The investigators recommended that these patients should be considered for pharmacotherapy.

Distal radial fractures often are the first clinical sign of osteoporosis because they tend to occur in younger patients compared with patients who sustain hip fractures. Studies have shown that patients who sustain distal radial fractures are more likely to be fully cognizant and independent, with effective neuromuscular control and walking speeds, because they are able to reach out and break their fall.[13] Hip and proximal humeral fractures, however, tend to occur in less functional patients who are unable to break their fall, resulting in impact on the shoulder or hip. Current evidence suggests that osteoporosis and poor BMD correlate with increasing severity

of the distal radial fractures, with more severe fractures leading to early and late displacement, late carpal malalignment, and malunion.[14]

DIAGNOSIS

Distal radial fractures also may be the first opportunity to evaluate and treat osteoporosis to reduce the risk of future fragility fractures.[1,15,16] A prospective, randomized controlled study showed that initiation of an osteoporosis workup by an orthopedic surgeon results in a statistically significant increase in treatment compared with referral to a primary care physician.[1] Treatment of osteoporosis should be initiated if it is a new diagnosis.

Because distal radial fractures may be the initial presentation of osteoporosis, the ability to diagnose osteoporosis accurately using hand and wrist radiographs would be helpful in expediting referral and initiating treatment; however, 1 study found that digital hand radiographs had poor accuracy compared with dual-energy x-ray absorptiometry (DEXA) scans and had only fair agreement in diagnosing osteoporosis.[17] Another study demonstrated that the second metacarpal cortical percentage calculated from standard radiographs of the hand and wrist may have a role in accurately screening for osteopenia and osteoporosis.[18] Hounsfield unit measurements from distal radial CT scans also have been reported to identify patients who require further metabolic bone disease workup, referral, and initiation of osteoporosis treatment[19]; however, it is difficult to justify the higher radiation dose associated with CT imaging and, therefore, it may not be practical in the clinical setting. At the least, a simple observation of thinned distal radial cortices on plain radiographs should prompt further evaluation with DEXA and medical management, given that the average radial bicortical thickness statistically correlates with femoral bone density.[20]

TREATMENT
Medical Treatment
Medical treatment can include vitamin D, calcium, bisphosphonate medications, and recombinant human parathyroid hormone (PTH), also known as teriparatide.

The effect of bisphosphonates on healing after distal radial fractures has been investigated because they often are used as the initial treatment of osteoporosis by inhibiting osteoclasts and decreasing bone resorption. One study found that early initiation of bisphosphonate treatment did not affect fracture healing or clinical outcomes of distal radial fractures.[21] In another study, patients receiving bisphosphonates at the time of sustaining a distal radial fracture had clinical outcomes similar to patients who were not receiving treatment.[22]

Bisphosphonates seem safe and can be continued throughout nonsurgical treatment of distal radial fractures without detrimental effects on healing or function.

Teriparatide, a recombinant form of PTH, contains the active terminal portion (1–34 amino residues) and recently has been shown to increase skeletal mass and bone strength and augment healing.[23–25] Teriparatide was Food and Drug Administration approved in 2002 for treatment of postmenopausal women and osteoporotic men who are at high risk of fracture. Teriparatide is administered daily by subcutaneous injection; treatment duration of more than 2 years is not recommended during a patient's lifetime. The daily dosing schedule simulates pulsatile PTH signaling, which leads to increased bone formation. In contrast, continuous infusion or constant PTH signaling would lead to bone resorption. Complications of teriparatide treatment include transient hypercalcemia, nausea, and headaches. It is contraindicated in patients with Paget disease and prior high radiation exposure because of concerns for a possible increased risk of osteosarcoma.[26] The true effectiveness of this medication in reducing fragility fracture is only beginning to be studied. A recent retrospective observational analysis found teriparatide most effective at 6 months after initiation of treatment after any fragility fracture, with a relative risk reduction still present at 2 years after discontinuation of treatment.[27]

Closed Reduction and Casting/Splinting

Nonoperative treatment can be considered for distal radial fragility fractures that are minimally displaced or are extra-articular and in which acceptable radiographic alignment can be maintained with immobilization after closed reduction. Fractures in patients who may be unfit for surgery, especially those with low functional demands, also may be treated conservatively. The benefits of closed treatment include minimizing the risk of infection, anesthesia, and surgical complications. Short-arm cast or splint immobilization often is required for 6 weeks to 8 weeks, with frequent follow-up to monitor for late displacement, angulation, or subsidence that can occur as a result of poor bone quality. One study reported that closed treatment of distal radial fractures in patients with osteoporosis increases the risk of dorsal and radial tilt resulting

in malunion.[28] Calcaneal BMD measurements may have some benefit in identifying patients at risk for severe malunion, but current evidence does not suggest a correlation between functional outcomes and BMD for conservatively treated distal radial fractures.[28,29] This may be because maintenance of anatomic alignment and reduction has not been shown to be essential for obtaining acceptable functional outcomes. Gutiérrez-Monclus and colleagues[30] found no significant correlation between acceptable alignment (according to radiological parameters) and short-term or medium-term functional outcomes in patients older than 60 with extra-articular distal radial fractures treated conservatively.

Operative Treatment

Current evidence and the most recent AAOS clinical guidelines comparing conservative and surgical treatment of distal radial fragility fractures are inconclusive and are limited by the use of a variety of functional outcome scores and an inability to compare a uniform fracture characteristic among all studies. A systematic review and meta-analysis did not demonstrate superior clinical outcomes after operative treatment in elderly patients with distal radial fractures[31]; however, the review did demonstrate that operative treatment can lead to better radiographic outcomes and grip strength compared with nonoperative treatment, despite an increased risk of complications. Another systematic review showed similar functional outcomes, using the Disabilities of the Arm, Shoulder and Hand (DASH) score, between operative and nonoperative treatment of distal radial fractures in the elderly.[32] A 2017 study comparing open reduction and internal fixation (ORIF) with volar locking plates to nonoperative treatment showed no difference in overall functional outcomes (DASH and Mayo wrist scores) at 12 months after injury.[33] The investigators did caution that longer follow-up is needed to determine if posttraumatic arthritis would negatively affect functional outcome scores. In contrast to this study, a 2018 randomized prospective study found that fixation led to better outcomes than conservative treatment in elderly patients with intra-articular distal radial fractures.[34] Finally, to minimize the risk associated with the use of anesthesia in the elderly population, wide-awake local anesthesia, no tourniquet, also has been described for treatment of distal radial fractures in patients with extensive comorbidities.[35] Well-designed, high level of evidence studies will help determine if there is any true benefit of surgical fixation considering the risks associated with anesthesia and surgery.

Kirschner wire fixation

K-wire fixation is a cost-effective method for stabilizing distal radial fractures. Percutaneous placement can minimize the risks associated with open surgery, but loss of fixation, subsidence, pin loosening, and infection can occur. In addition, K-wire removal often is recommended after fracture healing and can sometimes require a second procedure in the operating room. K-wire fixation may not be effective for fractures with comminution and significant shortening. One study demonstrated that K-wire fixation was effective in maintaining sagittal plane angulation after reduction but not radial length in extra-articular fragility fractures.[36] The best predictor of radial length was the radial length before fracture reduction, and the investigators recommended that K-wire fixation should not be used if radial shortening is visible on injury radiographs. Another study compared volar locking plate fixation to K-wire fixation and found that patients treated with volar locking plates had better functional outcomes in the early postoperative period and a reduced risk of developing complex regional pain syndrome.[37] The study also compared K-wire fixation to nonsurgical treatment and found a significantly higher percentage of excellent and good results, indicating that there may be a role for K-wire fixation over closed treatment.

Volar plating

The widespread use of volar locking plates for distal radial fractures is likely due to their ability to provide a strong biomechanical construct while using the familiar volar approach for most distal radial injury patterns, even in the presence of dorsal angulation and poor bone quality (**Fig. 1**).[34,38–40] Many studies have demonstrated the biomechanical strength of volar locking plates, with a recent study providing further evidence that osteoporosis and cortical thickness of the distal radius does not affect clinical outcomes after volar locking plate fixation.[39] Another benefit of volar locking plate fixation is earlier mobilization compared with cast treatment, with recent evidence suggesting that postoperative splinting and immobilization after volar locking plate fixation is unnecessary and even detrimental.[41] Flexion/extension, pronation/supination, pain and QuickDASH scores at 3 months after surgery were all better in the group without postoperative splinting.

Early studies questioned the capabilities of volar locking plates to provide improved functional outcomes in patients with osteoporosis. One study suggested that osteoporosis had a negative impact on functional outcomes in women treated with ORIF compared with women with osteopenia.[42] Another study suggested that osteoporosis had a negative effect on the range of motion of the wrist.[43] They found that activities of daily living were significantly restricted after plate osteosynthesis, despite finding no radiological difference between the osteoporotic and nonosteoporotic patients. In retrospect, the mean ages in the 2 groups were 56.5 years for the osteoporotic group compared with 37.1 years for the nonosteoporotic group, and this may have confounded their results. More recent studies have provided evidence supporting favorable functional outcomes, regardless of the presence of osteoporosis, after volar plate fixation of distal radial fragility fractures.[37,44,45] Several studies have shown that elderly patients, even those older than 70 years of age, treated with volar locking plate fixation have improved Mayo wrist scores and grip strength with no residual pain in most patients.[40,46] Another study showed that, despite loss of reduction for volar tilt and radial height within the first 4 months, the volar locking plate maintained intra-articular fracture stability with radiographic parameters within a functional range over time in most elderly patients (mean follow-up of 31 months).[45] There also is no clear association between BMD status and the risk of mechanical failure after volar locking plate fixation.[47]

Complications of volar plating

The complications associated with solar locking plates should be strongly considered (and discussed with patients preoperatively) when choosing surgical fixation.[2] One study reported an overall complication rate of 14.6% at 3.2-year follow-up of 576 patients who had volar plating.[48] Complications included carpal tunnel syndrome or change in sensibility, tendon irritation and rupture, deep infection, and complex regional pain syndrome. Another study reported a 7.5% complication rate in 824 patients. Application of the volar locking plate distal to the watershed line can increase the risk of flexor tendon irritation and rupture. Dorsal screw prominence also can lead to extensor tendon irritation or rupture.[49] A unique complication associated with the use of the volar locking plate is the occurrence of a longitudinal fracture line beneath the plate and extending proximally.[50,51]

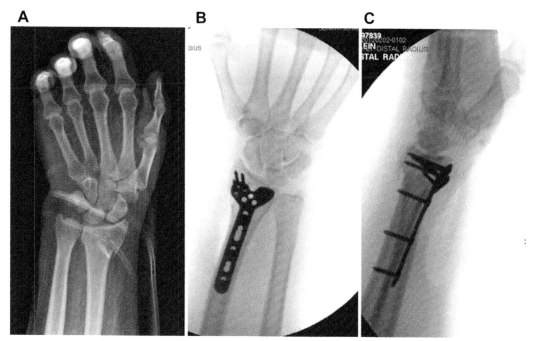

Fig. 1. (*A–C*) Volar plate fixation of a fracture of the distal radius. (*From* Perez EA. Fractures of the shoulder, arm, and forearm. In: Azar FM, Beaty JH, Canale ST, editors. Campbell's operative orthopaedics. 13th edition. Philadelphia: Elsevier; 2017. p. 2999; with permission.)

The fracture likely occurs after reduction of the plate to the bone with a nonlocking screw, followed by over-penetration of the near cortex by the conical head of a diaphyseal locking screw. This screw acts as a wedge, causing the longitudinal fracture line. Elderly patients may be more at risk because the near cortex may become more brittle with age and bone thinning.

Dorsal Plating

The use of dorsal plate fixation has decreased with increasing evidence supporting the ability of volar locking plate to provide stability for dorsally angulated distal radial fractures, familiarity of the volar approach to the distal radius, and early high rate of complications reported with dorsal plate fixation. There are certain fracture patterns, however, that may benefit from dorsal fixation and/or a dorsal approach for visualization and reduction. These patterns include dorsal shear fractures (dorsal Barton), die-punch fracture, and patterns in which indirect reduction cannot be obtained from a volar approach.[52] The most notable complication associated with dorsal plate fixation is attritional extensor tendon irritation and rupture. Most of these complications occurred in older-generation plates, with more recent studies reporting that favorable outcomes and minimal complications occur with newer-generation implants.[53–56] Newer dorsal implants can minimize attritional wear by having precontoured plates available in a variety of sizes with polished surfaces, tapered edges, and low-profile screw heads.[57] Similar to the volar locking plate, dorsal locking plates are available to improve fixation in osteoporotic bone and to allow early range of motion.

Fragment-specific Fixation

Fracture-specific fixation allows for a systematic approach for treatment of complex distal radial fractures by stabilizing each fragment individually to restore the radial and intermediate columns of the distal radius.[58] Various implants are designed to provide anatomic rigid fixation to the radial styloid, volar, and dorsal ulnar corner and articular shear fragments. Multiple incisions are often needed to obtain proper exposure if multiple fragments require fixation. Biomechanical studies demonstrate that applying an implant in more than 1 plane increases rigidity and the use of two 2.0-mm implants with a 50° to 90° offset angle between them in the axial plane provides stronger fixation than a single 3.5-mm plate.[59,60] A biomechanical cadaver study found significantly less linear displacement and angulation at the osteotomy site in the fragment-specific fixation group compared with volar locking plate at loads expected to be encountered during postoperative rehabilitation.[61] Angulation at the osteotomy site was significantly less, however, in the volar locking plate group at higher loads. Fragment-specific fixation can be used in conjunction with volar locking plate to provide biomechanically superior strength and stability if a stronger construct is required. Fracture-specific implants have the ability to stabilize volar rim fragments[62] and the volar ulnar corner while minimizing the risk for flexor tendon damage or rupture, a complication that can result from implant prominence due to restrictions of a larger fixed-angle device.[63] Stabilizing this fragment is essential to avoid the catastrophic complication of volar subluxation of the carpus.[64]

Outcomes of Fragment-specific Fixation

Benson and colleagues[65] reported good to excellent results with range of motion, grip strength, radiographic alignment and satisfaction scores in patients with intra-articular distal radius fractures treated with fragment-specific fixation. A randomized controlled study compared fragment-specific fixation to volar locking plates and demonstrated good results in both groups and similar patient-reported outcomes.[66] There was, however, a significantly higher complication rate for the fragment-specific group. There is clearly a role for fracture-specific implants because they allow

versatility and the ability to stabilize fractures that cannot be adequately treated with a single implant.[67-69]

Percutaneous Endomedullary Internal Fixation

Solarino and colleagues[70] investigated the use of the Epibloc system, a percutaneous endomedullary internal fixation system developed in Italy, in low-functioning patients with multiple medical comorbidities who would not respond well to the stress of extensive surgery. They compared the Epibloc system to volar locked plating and reported that volar locked plating was associated with better outcomes in both intra-articular and extra-articular distal radial fractures; however, in both the plating and Epibloc groups, grip strength mean values were greater than the minimal level needed to be considered a functional wrist. As a result, these investigators advocated the use of the Epibloc system in patients in whom minimally invasive surgery is preferred.

Intramedullary Fixation

Intramedullary fixation can be used selectively to treat dorsally angulated extra-articular and simple intra-articular distal radial fractures. The implant is inserted through the radial styloid, between the first and second dorsal compartments, using a limited dorsal radial incision (Fig. 2). Intramedullary fixation should be

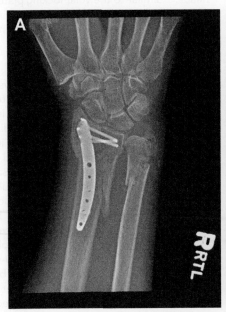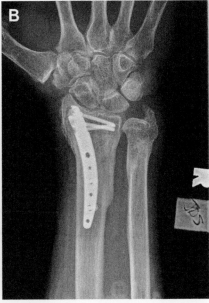

Fig. 2. (A) Three-week follow-up of a distal radial fracture with metaphyseal extension treated with an intramedullary nail. (B) Six-month follow-up radiograph shows union of the fracture. (From Harreld K, Li Z. Intramedullary fixation of distal radius fractures. Hand Clin 2010;26(3):367; with permission.)

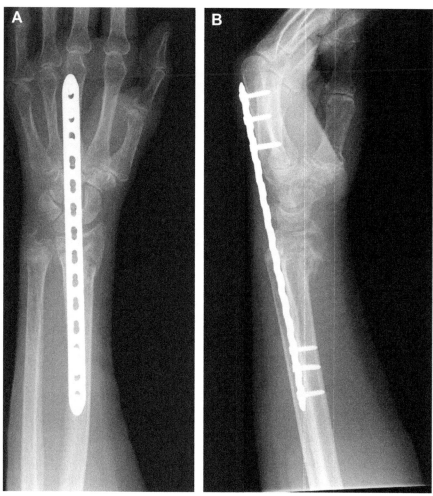

Fig. 3. Immediate postoperative (A) posteroanterior and (B) lateral radiographs demonstrate placement of a 14-hole, small-fragment locking compression plate, with 3 bicortical screws in the radial diaphysis and 3 in the third metacarpal. (*From* Richard MJ, Katolik LI, Hanel DP, et al. Distraction plating for the treatment of highly comminuted distal radius fractures in elderly patients. J Hand Surg Am 2012;37(5):951; with permission.)

avoided if the fracture cannot be preliminarily reduced by closed or percutaneous means because the implant cannot facilitate reduction, unlike a volar locking plate.[71] Marginal rim or sagittal shear intra-articular fracture fragments also cannot be adequately treated using an intramedullary implant. Advantages of intramedullary fixation include minimizing surgical exposure, preventing tendon irritation, and speeding return to activity.[72] Biomechanically, intramedullary fixation provides enough stability to allow for early postoperative range of motion through a load sharing, fixed-angle device.[73] A prospective case series demonstrated at least 90% return of wrist flexion, extension, ulnar deviation, radial deviation, pronation, supination, and grip strength compared with the contralateral side after intramedullary fixation in these fractures.[74]

When using the modified Mayo wrist score, there were 20 excellent and 9 good results. The study did not compare intramedullary fixation to other treatment options, such as the volar locking plate. Complications reported after intramedullary fixation include carpal tunnel syndrome, superficial radial nerve injury, screw loosening, and a proud screw tip that contacted the ulnar head.[72] Radial shortening with excessive volar tilt occurred in 2 distal radial fractures in the Nishiwaki and colleagues[74] study. The intramedullary construct can provide sufficient stability to prevent dorsal displacement[73,75]; however, it may be less effective in preventing volar displacement. Careful attention should be made to select an implant of appropriate size in patients with osteoporosis and a large intramedullary canal.[76]

Spanning Internal and External Fixation

Dorsal distraction plating (functioning as an internal fixator) has been described for treatment of highly comminuted intra-articular distal radial fractures and fractures in multiply injured patients. The technique varies in the literature, with some investigators fixing the plate to the second metacarpal (through the second dorsal compartment) and others to the third metacarpal (through the fourth dorsal compartment).[77] Dorsal distraction plating allows early weight bearing by spanning the radiocarpal joint, enabling a multiply injured patient to sit up, transfer, and ambulate without restriction (Fig. 3).[78] The implant usually is removed after 3 months, when fracture healing is complete. Hanel and colleagues[79] reported minor and major complication rates of 4.6% and 8.5%, respectively. Because plate fracture and screw failure occurred when a 2.7-mm plate and 2.4-mm screws were used, they recommended the use of a larger 3.5-mm plate and 2.7-mm screws. Other reported complications of dorsal plate distraction include finger stiffness requiring tenolysis, extensor tendon irritation, metacarpal fractures through a distal screw hole prior to plate removal, and 1 reported case of extensor tendon rupture after the patient did not return for planned plate removal.[79–82] The metacarpal fractures were treated closed and were healed by the time of plate removal. The current evidence for dorsal distraction plating is limited to retrospective case series, and there are no data comparing the technique to external fixation or plate fixation. Multiply injured patients often are younger than patients with osteoporotic distal radial fractures, with most dorsal distraction plating studies reporting an average age in the early fifties.[79] Evidence supporting the use of dorsal distraction plating for highly comminuted fractures in the elderly is yet to be determined.

Indications for external fixation are similar to dorsal distraction plating, with the notable additional indications of grossly contaminated wounds and significant soft tissue injury. External fixation avoids placement of an incision in these areas and can be used as temporary or definitive treatment. Evidence supporting the use of external fixators specifically for osteoporotic distal radial fragility fractures also is currently limited.

Wrist Hemiarthroplasty

Primary wrist hemiarthroplasty for irreparable distal radial fractures has been described in independent elderly patients (more than 65 years of age), with acceptable outcomes at 30-month follow-up.[78] A cement-less stemmed implant is instrumented into the distal radius with careful attention made to restore distal radial length. Irreparable fractures have been defined as any fracture that displays a combination of the criteria: AO type C complete intra-articular fracture, high extra-articular and intra-articular displacement scores, main fracture line distal to the watershed line, impaction, and circumferential comminution.[78] The main advantage of wrist hemiarthroplasty is early mobilization without the usual restrictions associated with concerns for implant failure and fracture healing. Future studies are required to determine long-term outcomes, implant survival rates, and late complications to fully validate this treatment option.

SUMMARY

Osteoporosis is a significant risk factor for distal radial fragility fractures in elderly patients. Good functional outcomes can be obtained with nonsurgical and surgical fixation methods, depending on the fracture configuration and patient age, comorbidities, activity level, and osteoporosis severity.

REFERENCES

1. Rozental TD, Makhni EC, Day CS, et al. Improving evaluation and treatment for osteoporosis following distal radial fractures. A prospective randomized intervention. J Bone Joint Surg Am 2008;90(5):953–61.

2. Pajarinen J, Lindahl J, Michelsson O, et al. Pertrochanteric femoral fractures treated with a dynamic hip screw or a proximal femoral nail. A randomized study comparing post-operative rehabilitation. J Bone Joint Surg Br 2005;87(1):76–81.

3. Rogmark C, Johnell O. Primary arthroplasty is better than internal fixation of displaced femoral neck fractures: a meta-analysis of 14 randomized studies with 2,289 patients. Acta Orthop 2006; 77(3):359–67.

4. Shauver MJ, Zhong L, Chung KC. Mortality after distal radial fractures in the Medicare population. J Hand Surg Eur Vol 2015;40(8):805–11.

5. Lauritzen JB, Schwarz P, McNair P, et al. Radial and humeral fractures as predictors of subsequent hip, radial or humeral fractures in women, and their seasonal variation. Osteoporos Int 1993;3(3):133–7.

6. Dewan N, MacDermid JC, Grewal R, et al. Risk factors predicting subsequent falls and osteoporotic fractures at 4 years after distal radius fractures—a prospective cohort study. Arch Osteoporos 2018; 13(1):32.

7. Rozenthal TD, Herder LM, Walley KC, et al. 25-hydroxyvitamin-D and bone turnover marker levels in patients with distal radial fractures. J Bone Joint Surg Am 2015;97(20):1685–93.

8. Saarelainen J, Hassi S, Honkanen R, et al. Bone loss and wrist fractures after withdrawal of hormone therapy: the 15-year follow-up of the OSTPRE cohort. Maturitas 2016;94:49–55.

9. Nellans KW, Kowalski E, Chung KC. The epidemiology of distal radius fractures. Hand Clin 2012; 28(2):113–25.

10. Xu W, Ni C, Yu R, et al. Risk factors for distal radius fracture in postmenopausal women. Orthopade 2017;46(5):447–50.

11. Øyen J, Brudvik C, Gjesdal CG, et al. Osteoporosis as a risk factor for distal radial fractures: a case-control study. J Bone Joint Surg Am 2011;93(4): 348–56.

12. Beattie K, Addachi J, Ioannidis G, et al. Estimating osteoporotic fracture risk following a wrist fracture: a tale of two systems. Arch Osteoporos 2015;10:13.

13. Vogt MT, Cauley JA, Tomaino MM, et al. Distal radius fractures in older women: a 10-year follow-up study of descriptive characteristics and risk factors. The study of osteoporotic fractures. J Am Geriatr Soc 2002;50(1):97–103.

14. Clayton RA, Gaston MS, Ralston SH, et al. Association between decreased bone mineral density and severity of distal radial fractures. J Bone Joint Surg Am 2009;91(3):613–9.

15. Padegimas EM, Osei DA. Evaluation and treatment of osteoporotic distal radius fractures in the elderly patient. Curr Rev Musculoskelet Med 2013;6(1): 41–6.

16. Sarfani S, Scrabeck T, Keams AE, et al. Clinical efficacy of a fragility care program in distal radius fracture patients. J Hand Surg Am 2014;39(4):664–9.

17. Miller AJ, Jones C, Liss F, et al. Qualitative evaluation of digital hand x-rays is not a reliable method to assess bone mineral density. Arch Bone Jt Surg 2017;5(1):10–3.

18. Schreiber JJ, Kamal RN, Yao J. Simple assessment of global done density and osteoporosis screening using standard radiographs of the hand. J Hand Surg Am 2017;42(4):244–9.

19. Schreiber JJ, Gausden EB, Anderson PA, et al. Opportunistic osteoporosis screening – gleaning additional information from diagnostic wrist CT scans. J Bone Joint Surg Am 2015;97(13):1095–100.

20. Webber T, Patel SP, Pensak M, et al. Correlation between distal radial cortical thickness and bone mineral density. J Hand Surg Am 2015;40(3):493–9.

21. Gong HS, Song CH, Lee YH, et al. Early initiation of bisphosphonate does not affect healing and outcomes of volar plate fixation of osteoporotic distal radial fractures. J Bone Joint Surg Am 2012;94(19): 1729–36.

22. Shoji KE, Earp BE, Rozental RD. The effect of bisphosphonates on the clinical and radiographic outcomes of distal radius fractures in woman. J Hand Surg Am 2018;43(2):115–22.

23. Collinge C, Favela J. Use of teriparatide in osteoporotic fracture patients. Injury 2016;47(Suppl 1): S36–8.

24. Im GI, Lee SH. Effect of teriparatide on healing of atypical femoral fractures: a systemic review. J Bone Metab 2015;22(4):183–9.

25. Neer RM, Leder BZ, Burnett SM, et al. Effects of teriparatide, alendronate, or both on bone turnover in osteoporotic men. J Clin Endocrinol Metab 2006; 91(8):2882–7.

26. Subbiah V, Madsen VS, Raymond AK, et al. Of mice and men: divergent risks of teriparatide-induced osteosarcoma. Osteoporos Int 2010;21(6):1041–5.

27. Boytsov N, Zhang X, Surihara T, et al. Osteoporotic fractures and associated hospitalizations among patients treated with teriparatide compared to a matched cohort of patients not treated with teriparatide. Curr Med Res Opin 2015;31(9):1665–75.

28. Brogren E, Petranek M, Atroshi I. Cast-treated distal radius fractures: a prospective cohort study of radiological outcomes and their association with impaired calcaneal bone mineral density. Arch Orthop Trauma Surg 2015;135(7):927–33.

29. Boymans TA, van Helden S, Kessels A, et al. Bone mineral density is not correlated with one-year functional outcome in distal radial fractures: a preliminary study. Eur J Trauma Emerg Surg 2009; 35(3):281–6.

30. Gutiérrez-Monclus R, Gutiérrez-Espinoza H, Zavala-González J, et al. Correlation between radiological parameters and functional outcomes in patients older than 60 years of age with distal radius fractures. Hand (N Y) 2018. 1558944718770203. [Epub ahead of print].

31. Chen Y, Chen X, Li Z, et al. Safety and efficacy of operative versus nonsurgical management of distal radius fractures in elderly patients: a systematic review and meta-analysis. J Hand Surg Am 2016; 41(3):404–13.

32. Ju JH, Jin GZ, Li GX, et al. Comparison of treatment outcomes between nonsurgical and surgical treatment of distal radius fracture in elderly: a systematic review and meta-analysis. Langenbecks Arch Surg 2015;400(7):767–79.

33. Toon DH, Premchandd RAX, Sim J, et al. Outcomes and financial implications of intra-articular distal radius fractures: a comparative study of open reduction internal fixation (ORIF) with volar locking plates versus nonoperative management. J Orthop Traumatol 2017;18(3):229–34.

34. Martinez-Mendez D, Lizaur-Utrilla A, de-Juan-Herrero J. Intra-articular distal radius fractures in elderly patients: a randomized prospective study

of casting versus volar plating. J Hand Surg Eur Vol 2018;43(2):142–7.

35. Ahmad AA, Yi LM, Ahmad AR. Plating of distal radius fracture using the wide-awake anesthesia technique. J Hand Surg Am 2018. https://doi.org/10.1016/j.jhsa.2018.03.033.

36. Kennedy C, Kennedy MT, Niall D, et al. Radiological outcomes of distal radius extra-articular fragility fractures treated with extra-focal kirschner wires. Injury 2010;41(6):639–42.

37. Tomaszuk M, Kiryluk J, Tomaszuk A, et al. Evaluation of treatment of low-energy distal radial fractures in postmenopausal women. Ortop Traumatol Rehabil 2017;19(1):55–65.

38. Ballal A, Sadasivan AK, Hegde A, et al. Open reduction and volar plate fixation of dorsally displaced distal radius fractures: a prospective study of functional and radiological outcomes. J Clin Diagn Res 2016;10(12):RC01–4.

39. Lee JI, Park KC, Joo IH, et al. The effect of osteoporosis on the outcomes after volar locking plate fixation in female patients older than 50 years with unstable distal radius fractures. J Hand Surg Am 2018;43(8):731–7.

40. Shimura H, Nimura A, Fujita K, et al. Mid-term functional outcome after volar locking plate fixtation of distal radius fractures in elderly patients. J Hand Surg Asian Pac Vol 2018;23(2):238–42.

41. Duprat A, Diaz JJH, Vernet P, et al. Volar locking plate fixation of distal radius fractures: splint versus immediate mobilization. J Wrist Surg 2018;7(3):237–42.

42. Fitzpatrick SK, Casemyr NE, Zurakowski D, et al. The effect of osteoporosis on outcomes of operatively treated distal radius fractures. J Hand Surg Am 2012;37(1):2027–34.

43. Büyükkurt CD, Bülbul M, Ayanoglu S, et al. The effects of osteoporosis on functional outcome in patients with distal radius fracture treated with plate osteosynthesis. Acta Orthop Traumatol Turc 2012;46(2):89–95.

44. Choi WS, Lee HJ, Kim DY, et al. Does osteoporosis have a negative effect on the functional outcome of an osteoporotic distal radial fracture treated with a volar locking plate? Bone Joint J 2015;97-B(2):229–34.

45. Martinez-Mendez D, Lizaur-Itrilla A, de Juan-Herrero J. Prospective study of comminuted articular distal radius fracture stabilized by volar plating in the elderly. Int Orthop 2018;42(9):2243–8.

46. Piuzzi NS, Zaidenberg EE, Duarte MP, et al. Volar plate fixation in patients older than 70 years with AO type C distal radial fractures: clinical and radiologic outcomes. J Wrist Surg 2017;6(3):194–200.

47. Daniel R, Joerg G, Kurt K, et al. The effect of local bone mineral density on the rate of mechanical failure after surgical treatment of distal radius fractures: a prospective multicenter cohort study including 249 patients. Arch Orthop Trauma Surg 2015;135(2):201–7.

48. Thorninger R, Madsen ML, Waever D, et al. Complications of volar locking plating of distal radius fractures in 576 patients with 3.2 years follow-up. Injury 2017;48(6):1104–9.

49. Satake H, Hanaka N, Honma R, et al. Complications of distal radius fractures treated by volar locking plate fixation. Orthopedics 2016;39(5):e893–6.

50. Otremski H, Dolkart O, Atlan F, et al. Hairline fractures following volar plating of the distal radius: a recently recognized hardware-related complication. Skeletal Radiol 2018;47(6):833–7.

51. Sügün TS, Gürbüz Y, Özaksar K, et al. A new complication in volar locking plating of the distal radius: longitudinal fractures of the near cortex. Acta Orthop Traumatol Turc 2016;50(2):147–52.

52. Lutsky K, Boyer M, Goldfarb C. Dorsal locked plate fixation of distal radius fractures. J Hand Surg Am 2013;38(7):1414–22.

53. Kamath AF, Zurakowski D, Day CS. Low-profile dorsal plating for dorsally angulated distal radius fractures: an outcomes study. J Hand Surg Am 2006;31(7):1061–7.

54. Ring D, Jupiter JB, Brennwalk J, et al. Prospective multicenter trial of a plate for dorsal fixation of distal radius fractures. J Hand Surg Am 1997;22(5):777–84.

55. Rozental TD, Beredjiklian PK, Bozentka DJ. Functional outcome and complications following two types of dorsal plating for unstable fractures of the distal part of the radius. J Bone Joint Surg Am 2003;85(10):1956–60.

56. Yu JK. Complications of low-profile dorsal versus volar locking plates in the distal radius: a comparative study. J Hand Surg Am 2011;36(7):1135–41.

57. Tavakolian JD, Jupiter JB. Dorsal plating for distal radius fractures. Hand Clin 2005;21(3):341–6.

58. Leslie B, Medoff RJ. Fracture specific fixation of distal radius fractures. Tech Orthop 2000;15:336–52.

59. Dodds SD, Cornelissen S, Jossan S, et al. A biomechanical comparison of fragment-specific fixation and augmented external fixation for intra-articular distal radius fractures. J Hand Surg Am 2002;27(6):953–64.

60. Peine R, Rikli DA, Hoffman R, et al. Comparison of three different plating techniques for the dorsum of the distal radius: a biomechanical study. J Hand Surg Am 2000;25(1):29–33.

61. Grindel SI, Wang M, Gerlach M, et al. Biomechanical comparison of fixed-angle volar plate versus fixed-angle volar plate plus fragment-specific fixation in a cadaveric distal radius fracture model. J Hand Surg Am 2007;32(2):194–9.

62. Bakker AJ, Shin AY. Fragment-specific volar hook plate for volar marginal rim fractures. Tech Hand Up Extrem Surg 2014;18(1):56–60.

63. Cross AW, Schmidt CC. Flexor tendon injuries following locked volar plating of distal radius fractures. J Hand Surg 2008;33(2):164–7.

64. Harness NG, Jupiter JB, Orbay JL, et al. Loss of fixation of the volar lunate facet fragment in fractures of the distal part of the radius. J Bone Joint Surg Am 2004;86(9):1900–8.

65. Benson LS, Minihane KP, Stern LD, et al. The outcome of intra-articular distal radius fractures treated with fragment-specific fixation. J Hand Surg Am 2006;31(8):1333–9.

66. Landgren M, Abramo A, Geijer M, et al. Fragment-specific fixation versus volar locking plates in primarily nonreducible or secondarily redisplaced distal radius fractures: a randomized controlled study. J Hand Surg Am 2017;42(3):156–65.

67. Brogan DM, Richard MJ, Ruck D, et al. Management of severely comminuted distal radius fractures. J Hand Surg 2015;40(9):1905–14.

68. Lam J, Wolfe SW. Distal radius fractures: what cannot be fixed with a volar plate?—the role of fragment-specific fixation in modern fracture treatment. Oper Tech Sports Med 2010;18:181–8.

69. Saw N, Roberts C, Cutbush K, et al. Early experience with the TriMed fragment-specific fracture fixation system in intraarticular distal radius fractures. J Hand Surg Eur Vol 2008;33(1):53–8.

70. Solarino G, Vicenti G, Abate A, et al. Volar locking plate vs epibloc system for distal radius fractures in the elderly. Injury 2016;47(Suppl 4):S84–90.

71. Harreld K, Li Z. Intramedullary fixation of distal radius fractures. Hand Clin 2010;26(3):263–372.

72. Falk SS, Mittlmeier T, Gradi G. Results of geriatric distal radius fractures treated by intramedullary fixation. Injury 2016;47(Suppl 7):S31–5.

73. Capo JT, Kinchelow T, Brooks T, et al. Biomechanical stability of four fixation constructs for distal radius fractures. Hand (N Y) 2009;4(3):272–8.

74. Nishiwaki M, Tazaki K, Shimizu H, et al. Prospective study of distal radial fractures treated with an intramedullary nail. J Bone Joint Surg Am 2011;93(15):1436–41.

75. Burkhart KJ, Nowak TE, Gradi G, et al. Intramedullary nailing vs. palmar locked plating for unstable dorsally comminuted distal radius fractures: a biomechanical study. Clin Biomech (Bristol, Avon) 2010;25(6):771–5.

76. Wakasugi T, Shirasaka R. Intramedullary nail fixation for displaced and unstable distal radial fractures in patients aged 65 years or older. J Hand Surg Asian Pac Vol 2016;32(1):k59–63.

77. Dahl J, Lee DJ, Elfar JC. Anatomic relationships in distal radius bridge plating: a cadaveric study. Hand (N Y) 2015;10($):657–62.

78. Huang JI, Peterson B, Bellevue K, et al. Biomehanical assessment of the dorsal spanning bridge plate in distal radius fracture fixation: implications for immediate weight bearing. Hand (N Y) 2018;13(3):336–40.

79. Hanel DP, Ruhlman SD, Katolik LI, et al. Complications associated with distraction plate fixation of wrist fractures. Hand Clin 2010;26(2):237–43.

80. Lewis S, Mostofi A, Stevanovic M, et al. Risk of tendon entrapment under a dorsal bridge plate in a distal radius fracture model. J Hand Surg Am 2015;40(3):500–4.

81. Matzon JL, Kenniston J, Berejiklian PK. Hardware-related complications after dorsal plating for displaced distal radius fractures. Orthopedics 2014;37(11):e978–82.

82. Herzberg G, Walch A, Burnier M. Wrist hemiarthroplasty for irreparable DRF in the elderly. Eur J Orthop Surg Traumatol 2018. https://doi.org/10.1007/s00590-018-2228-5.

Shoulder and Elbow

Surgical Considerations in the Treatment of Osteoporotic Proximal Humerus Fractures

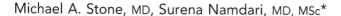

Michael A. Stone, MD, Surena Namdari, MD, MSc*

KEYWORDS

- Proximal humerus fracture • Fragility fracture • Osteoporosis • Osteopenia
- Open reduction internal fixation • Shoulder arthroplasty

KEY POINTS

- Open reduction internal fixation for proximal humerus fractures has a high complication rate.
- Several options exist for augmentation in cases of osteoporosis.
- Reverse total shoulder arthroplasty is becoming increasingly common for primary treatment of 3-part or 4-part fractures of the proximal humerus in the elderly.

INTRODUCTION

Proximal humerus fractures are the third most common fragility fracture type in elderly patients and can be a significant cause of morbidity and loss of function.[1,2] The incidence of proximal humerus fractures in Medicare patients from 1999 to 2005 was approximately 250 per 100,000 patients.[2] Eighty percent of those affected with proximal humerus fractures are women and aged between 80 and 89 years, with most operative cases falling in the 74-year to 84-year range.[1,2] Osteoporotic bone also significantly increases the risk for proximal humerus fractures, with the risk increasing 2.6 times greater in osteoporotic bone (12.1 per 1000 woman-years) compared with nonosteoporotic bone (4.6 per 1000 woman-years) in one study.[3]

The preponderance of these fractures in women and older patients is likely due to the association between these demographic factors and the diagnosis of osteoporosis or osteopenia. Poor bone quality can lead to comminution, thin cortical bone, and crushed cancellous bone that makes obtaining and maintaining a reduction and achieving adequate hardware fixation challenging. Treatment with locking plates has provided fixed-angle constructs with lower risks of screw back-out; however, challenges remain with treatment of patients with poor bone quality, such as varus collapse and screw cutout. A clearer understanding of predictors of fixation failure and the encouraging early results of reverse total shoulder arthroplasty (RTSA) have resulted in increased utilization of RTSA for the primary treatment of proximal humerus fractures. The purpose of this article was to review surgical technique considerations in the surgical treatment of proximal humerus fractures.

OPERATIVE VERSUS NONOPERATIVE TREATMENT

There is currently no widely accepted consensus on indications for surgical treatment of osteoporotic proximal humerus fractures. A recent

Disclosure Statement: Dr M.A. Stone has nothing to disclose. Dr S. Namdari receives research funding from Arthrex, Zimmer, Depuy-Synthes, and Integra LifeSciences; is a consultant for DJO Surgical and Miami Device Solutions; and receives royalties from DJO Surgical, Miami Device Solutions, and Elsevier.
Department of Orthopaedic Surgery, The Rothman Institute, Thomas Jefferson University, 925 Chestnut Street, 5th Floor, Philadelphia, PA 19107, USA
* Corresponding author.
E-mail address: Surena.Namdari@rothmaninstitute.com

randomized controlled trial showed no difference in outcomes between operative compared with nonoperative treatment of proximal humerus fractures.[4] Despite a high level of evidence, limitations of this study, including multiple surgeons, variable surgical techniques, and lack of radiographic evaluation, have made it difficult to draw firm conclusions.

In the case that a nonoperative treatment plan is initiated, passive motion of the shoulder is encouraged to start relatively early in the healing process. In our practice, passive range of motion exercises are started at 2 weeks from the date of the injury. Patients are advanced to active-assisted motion and active motion at 4 and 6 weeks postinjury, respectively. Strengthening is typically initiated between 8 and 12 weeks and is based on radiographic healing (Table 1).

In the absence of open or neurovascular injury, the indications for surgical treatment of proximal humerus fractures are controversial. Commonly, the same fracture pattern can be treated nonoperatively, with surgical fixation, or with arthroplasty, depending on multiple variables including patient age, medical comorbidities, activity level, and goals/expectations of treatment. The remaining sections focus on surgical considerations to improve fixation with locking plate constructs and to enhance replacement with RTSA. Although intramedullary nailing, percutaneous fixation, external fixation, nitinol cage fixation, and hemiarthroplasty are options for treatment, they are beyond the scope of this review.

Locking Plate Constructs

Plate fixation allows anatomic reduction and control of the fracture fragments, and can be performed via a deltopectoral or a deltoid splitting approach.[5] Traditionally, screw fixation in the poor metaphyseal bone of the proximal humerus has risked loss of fixation and screw back-out. Biomechanical studies have shown that decreasing bone density has a drastic effect on the holding strength of screws.[6] The advent of locked plating has allowed for the creation of screw constructs that remain in a fixed-angle position irrespective of bone quality.[7] Clinical results of locking plate fixation of proximal humerus fractures have demonstrated successful outcomes. A meta-analysis of locking plate fixation for proximal humerus fractures showed an average overall constant score of 74 with minimum 18-month follow-up, 79 for 2-part fractures, 72 for 3-part fractures, and 66 for 4-part fractures.[8] Despite the improvements in plate technology, complication and reoperation rates remain a concern.

Causes of complications are multifactorial, and involve patient-related factors (eg, comorbid conditions, smoking), fracture-specific factors (eg, bone quality, comminution, fracture pattern), surgical factors (eg, plate/screw placement, reduction quality), and postoperative rehabilitation. Varus malunion was the most common complication (16.3%) in a meta-analysis by Sproul and colleagues,[8] followed by avascular necrosis (AVN) (10.8%), screw cutout (7.5%), subacromial impingement (4.8%), and infection (3.5%). Screw cutout was the most common reason for revision surgery. Several other studies have reported a high rate of screw cutout as a common complication, with a rate ranging from 7% to 57%.[9–12] In a study at a tertiary referral center for proximal humerus fixation complications, AVN (68%), malunion (63%), and malreduction (55%) were the most common complications. Secondary screw cutout (57%) and glenoid destruction (44%) accounted for the most common implant-related complications.[10]

SURGICAL CONSIDERATIONS
Reduction Quality

Quality reduction is an important prognostic factor in the treatment of proximal humerus fractures with open reduction internal fixation (ORIF). Schnetzke and colleagues[13] showed that anatomic or near-anatomic reduction compared with malreduction in OTA type C fractures is associated with improved clinical outcome at a 3.1-year follow-up (constant score 65.4% vs 47.6%, respectively). Malreduction of the greater tuberosity >5 mm was associated with a threefold increased risk of complications,

Table 1			
Nonoperative treatment protocol			
Week 2	**Week 4**	**Week 6**	**Weeks 8–12**
Passive motion, including the Codman exercise	Active-assisted motion (FF, ER, IR)	Active motion (FF, ER, IR)	Strengthening (based on radiographic healing)

Abbreviations: ER, external rotation; FF, forward flexion; IR, internal rotation.

revisions, and inferior clinical outcomes measured by the constant score. Mild varus did not affect clinical outcomes; however, head-shaft displacement >5 mm resulted in a significantly poorer clinical outcome. Despite superior clinical outcomes with improved reduction, complications (32.7%) and revisions (27.6%) remained high in this series.

Plate/Screw Placement

Proximal or distal plate positioning is an important surgical consideration and is a surgeon-controlled variable that can influence subacromial impingement (**Fig. 1**). More distally placed plates are less likely to cause plate impingement against the acromion. Proximal plate placement can be a result of poor surgical technique, poor fracture reduction, or small proximal humeral dimensions. Although plates are available in variable lengths, the dimensions of the proximal portion of precontoured locking plates are typically one size. Because of this, patient-specific variability in proximal humeral dimensions can result in proximal plate placement. In fixed-angle locking plate designs, plate positioning also has a profound influence on screw positions. Polyaxial locking plate designs allow for greater freedom of screw placement irrespective of plate position.

Screw position is most important in the calcar. Placement of calcar screws is critical in metaphyseal comminution to achieve medial column support.[14–17] The placement of the calcar screws in a more distal position, as opposed to a more proximal position within the head, is critical for improved biomechanical stability.[18] Gardner and colleagues[14] originally described the importance of medial calcar support in cases of medial fracture comminution. Functional stability of the

medial column was considered restored if there was cortical contact with anatomic reduction, lateral impaction, or locking screws placed in the inferomedial proximal humeral head (calcar screws). Proximal humerus fixation without adequate medial support sustained 53% loss of reduction, whereas the medial support group had no failures. The investigators concluded medial support was critical in reducing varus collapse and malreduction.[14] Another recent study defined the optimal screw location for medial column support. Padegimas and colleagues[19] defined the optimal placement of the calcar screw to be within 12 mm of the calcar (calcar distance) and a calcar ratio of 25% (defined as the ratio of the calcar distance and humeral head diameter). These 2 measurements were shown to be strongly predictive of fixation failure. Adequately reduced fractures had an optimal threshold of 13.1 mm and 26.1%, whereas malreduced fractures had a lower threshold of 11.4 mm and 23.4% for the calcar distance and calcar ratio, respectively.

In a biomechanical study using 11 matched pairs of human cadaveric proximal humerus fractures, medial calcar comminution decreased the mean load to failure by 48% and energy to failure by 44%. The use of calcar screws increased the mean load to failure by 31% and energy to failure by 44%, underscoring the importance of calcar screw support in cases of medial comminution.[17]

Suture Augmentation

Suture augmentation of the tuberosities is performed with the proposed benefit of additional fixation of the tuberosities to the plate. Frequently, the bone of the tuberosities is of poor quality, and the sutures are placed at the

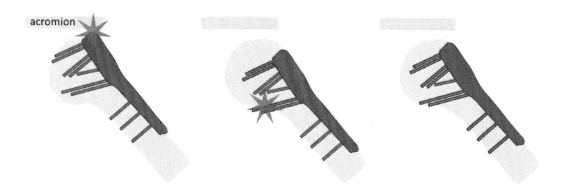

Too high - impingement   Too low – poor fixation   Appropriate height

Fig. 1. Effect of plate placement on subacromial impingement.

bone-tendon interface to prevent tendon tearing or pullout from the soft metaphyseal bone. Although this technique is frequently used in clinical practice, the data to support the use of suture augmentation is quite poor. A biomechanical study using a 3-part proximal humerus fracture model and locking plate constructs in cadavers showed no significant difference in interfragmentary strain with tagging sutures compared with no sutures.[20] This finding was confirmed in a more recent biomechanical study that added cyclic loading and load to failure, again with no statistically significant differences between groups.[21] Another biomechanical study using a 2-part fracture model failed to show any benefit of suture fixation as well.[22] One must bear in mind that the bone quality is frequently quite poor in a clinical setting and fragments may be impacted, resulting in suboptimal screw fixation; and so, the biomechanical testing conditions may not accurately replicate the clinical situation.

Bone Quality and Augmentation Assessment

Radiographs. Measurement of the bone density using standard radiographs of the shoulder is a useful preoperative technique to judge a patient's bone quality before discovery in the operating room. Tingart and colleagues[23] described a technique to judge bone density of the proximal humerus using cortical thickness of the medial and lateral cortices on anteroposterior view, with the first level measured at the most proximal level of the humeral diaphysis where the endosteal bone is parallel, and the second point 20 mm distal to this. The investigators determined that a combined cortical thickness of less than 4 mm was associated with significantly lower bone mineral density (BMD) than those humeri with greater than 4 mm.

Hepp and colleagues[24] measured the cortical index ([total area − bone marrow]/total area) in patients with a proximal humerus fracture at the level described by Bloom and colleagues,[25] and compared the cortical index to patients without a fracture in a matched-pairs analysis. The investigators found that the cortical index was significantly lower in the fracture group, but rate of reoperation was not statistically different between groups.

Computed tomography. Measurement of bone quality from computed tomography (CT) of the shoulder is usually readily available, as this imaging modality is frequently performed in anticipation for surgery. Krappinger and

colleagues[26] were the first to describe a technique to measure bone density of the proximal humerus using spiral CT scans. True axial cuts were taken at 3 equidistant levels in the proximal humerus and measured with Hounsfield Units. BMD measurements at the proximal humerus measured on CT correlated with measurements at various sites throughout the body, including lumbar spine, proximal femur, and forearm.

A more recent study compared the Krappinger technique with several other techniques using quantitative CT (QCT) and high-resolution peripheral CT. A measurement of the articular cap region bone mineral content using clinical QCT measurements showed the highest correlation to cyclic load to failure of the compared groups, including the Krappinger method.[27] This may be a useful new technique with improved accuracy as compared with conventional methods of measuring BMD.

Fibular strut allograft

Fibular strut allograft was first introduced for treatment of nonunions of the surgical neck of the proximal humerus as described by Walch and colleagues.[28] Subsequently, this technique has been modified for use in primary treatment of proximal humerus fractures.[29] This technique involves placing a fibular strut allograft within the intramedullary canal before placement of fixation. This has the advantage of creating a medial column of support in cases of severe metadiaphyseal comminution with the proposed benefit of preventing varus collapse of the humeral head (**Fig. 2**). Three biomechanical studies in human cadavers using a "gap model" to represent lack of medial column support, showed superior biomechanical stability when using the fibular strut compared with plate alone.[30–32] This technique may be most useful in cases of varus collapse, treatment of humeral nonunions, and cases of severe metadiaphyseal comminution.

Cancellous graft

Iliac crest autograft bone (ICBG) is another option for 4-part fractures with severe comminution. In a study of 21 patients with severe 4-part proximal humerus fractures, ICBG was used in addition to locking plate fixation with average 27-month follow-up. No cases of AVN occurred and union was achieved in 100% of shoulders. In another study using locked plating for 3-part and 4-part proximal humerus fractures, Ricchetti and colleagues[33] used cancellous bone allograft chips with demineralized bone matrix with minimum 6-month follow-up. The investigators

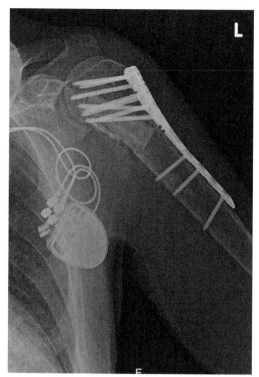

Fig. 2. Fibular strut allograft placed medially to restore calcar. Multiple locking screws placed in calcar.

reported complications in their cohort of 54 shoulders including 1 case of AVN, 5 patients who developed asymptomatic varus malunion, and 1 nonunion that healed after revision with ICBG.

Injectable calcium-based cements

Calcium phosphate cements may be used, as they can be injected as liquid and harden in vivo by normothermic crystallization. Calcium phosphate has the additional benefit of improved compressive strength and structural support. Kwon and colleagues[34] demonstrated improved stiffness using calcium phosphate cement across 3 fixation types in a cadaveric model. In a retrospective study of 92 acute proximal humerus fractures with metaphyseal defects, Egol and colleagues[35] showed significantly decreased fracture displacement and no evidence of intra-articular screw penetration when using calcium phosphate cement compared with cancellous chips or no augmentation with a mean follow-up of 16 months. Although these short-term results are encouraging, this study is limited by nonrandomization and lack of long-term follow-up.

The authors' preferred technique. In the senior author's practice, if an adequate reduction cannot be obtained based on the parameters discussed by Schnetzke and colleagues,[13] fixation is not performed, and strong consideration is given to arthroplasty. A polyaxial plate design is preferred to allow for the combination of distal plate position and optimal calcar screw position. Suture augmentation is routinely performed in cases of 3-part and 4-part fractures. Short and medially positioned fibular strut grafts are used in cases of osteoporotic 2-part fractures with calcar comminution, as these patterns are least likely to develop AVN, necessitating arthroplasty. When bone voids are encountered after reduction of 3-part or 4-part fractures, cancellous allograft chips are commonly used to improve fixation and prevent overreduction of the greater tuberosity into cavitary defects (Box 1).

Reverse total shoulder arthroplasty

Hemiarthroplasty has been the historical treatment for unreconstructible fractures of the proximal humerus.[36,37] This has changed over the recent years in favor of RTSA for the treatment of unreconstructible proximal humerus fractures in the elderly. The rate of RTSA for treatment of proximal humerus fractures has almost doubled from 2011 to 2013, rising from 13% of operative cases to 24% of operative cases, with hemiarthroplasty dropping from 28% to 21%.[38] Unlike hemiarthroplasty, RTSA does not necessitate tuberosity healing to achieve a successful result.[39,40] RTSA functions by 3 specific mechanisms: medializing the center of glenohumeral rotation; distalizing the center of rotation, which tensions the deltoid; and achieving a more constrained articulation, which allows the shear forces of shoulder abduction to be converted into a compressive force.

Complications related to RTSA include intraoperative fracture, component malposition, and nerve injury.[40] Postoperative complications include tuberosity failure, stiffness, instability, acromial stress fracture, scapular notching, and implant loosening.

Box 1
Open reduction internal fixation key points

1. Reduction quality is an important factor in postoperative outcomes

2. Medial column support is essential if medial comminution present, and can be achieved with anatomic reduction, or locked calcar screws

3. Augmentation to fixation can aid in reducing loss of fixation

SURGICAL CONSIDERATIONS
Stem Position/Fixation

The humeral stem should be positioned in such a way that diaphyseal fixation is optimized and anatomic fixation of the tuberosities to the implant is possible. Shortening of the humeral component can lead to instability if adequate soft tissue tension cannot be created.[41] Placing the cement in a proximal position can lead to overtensioning of the soft tissues and may lead to difficulty with implant reduction. In the setting of hemiarthroplasty, Murachovsky and colleagues[42] determined the distance between the upper border of the pectoralis major tendon insertion on the humerus and the top of the humeral head (averaged 5.6 cm). The investigators indicated that this distance is a useful landmark that will aid in accurate restoration of humeral length when reconstructing complex proximal humeral fractures. In cases of severe comminution, radiographs of the contralateral shoulder may help in determining length.[41,43]

Press-fit or cemented stems may be used in cases of proximal humerus fractures. When using a cemented stem, the cement is typically kept out of the metaphyseal region to not interfere with tuberosity healing. The stem may be cemented in place and cancellous bone can be used in the metaphyseal region as described by Formaini and colleagues.[44] There is currently no study directly comparing outcomes of cemented versus cementless stems in proximal humerus fractures; the outcomes of RTSA for other indications may be extrapolated.

Tuberosity Reduction and Fixation

Although greater tuberosity healing is not critical for a successful result, healing of the greater tuberosity in RTSA is important for improved external rotation (ER).[45] In a systematic review of RTSA for proximal humerus fractures in the elderly, forward elevation, ER at the side, and ER at 90° of abduction was significantly improved with a repaired tuberosity.[46] Gallinet and colleagues[47] compared outcomes of an anatomically healed tuberosity with those with malunion. The anatomically healed tuberosity group had significantly improved ER, Disabilities of Arm, Shoulder, and Hand (DASH) and constant scores compared with the malunion group. Appropriate tuberosity reduction and fixation can be challenging in the setting of bony comminution and local osteoporosis. A recent biomechanical study showed less tuberosity interfragmentary rotation when using cerclage cable as compared with suture fixation. This study, however, used cadaveric shoulders with a higher BMD than typically seen in severely osteoporotic shoulders.[48]

Grafting of the tuberosities should be performed whenever possible to improve healing. In one clinical study, tuberosity grafting with humeral head block autograft improved rates of tuberosity healing and clinical outcome scores at mean follow-up of 16 months. Tuberosity union was achieved in 78% (14/18) of patients in the grafting group, and 40% (6/15) of patients in the nongrafted group. Improved strength and clinical outcome scores, including the DASH and American Shoulder and Elbow Surgeons scores, were attributed to a higher tuberosity healing rate in the grafted group.[49] Another study using the "black and tan" technique, in which the stem is cemented into the diaphysis and cancellous graft is used at the metaphyseal region, reported healing rates were 88%.[44] Levy and Badman[50] advocated for maximizing surface contact area with the tuberosity using a "horseshoe graft" fashioned from the humeral head, demonstrating a healing rate of 86%.

The authors' preferred technique

The senior author judges stem position by measuring the amount of calcar bone attached to the fractured humeral head segment. If there is no bone attached to the head segment, the stem is positioned flush with the medial aspect of the humerus. If there is bone attached to the humeral head or metaphyseal comminution, the bone is measured with a ruler and the stem height is adjusted. Utilization of cement is based on the quality of the press-fit achieved intraoperatively. Bone from the humeral head is commonly impaction grafted into the humeral shaft to maximize a press-fit. When cement is used, a cement restrictor is placed distally, and cement is commonly pressurized into the humeral shaft in cases of metaphyseal comminution or poor bone quality. With regard to greater tuberosity reduction, the tuberosity is commonly malreduced in a distal position due to aggressive vertical compression. An appropriate "read" of the anatomic tuberosity position often can be observed at the lateral aspect of the humerus and the distal aspect of the greater tuberosity (Fig. 3). Multiple nonabsorbable sutures are placed at the bone-tendon interface of each fragment to achieve both horizontal and vertical fixation. A minimum of 2 heavy, nonabsorbable sutures are placed through the

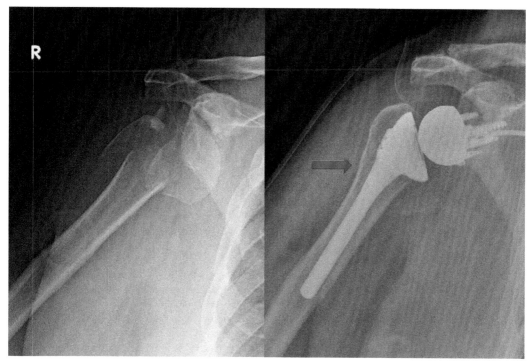

Fig. 3. Press-fit reverse for fracture-dislocation with tuberosity reduction and appropriate stem height shown. Reduction of greater tuberosity fragment (*arrow*).

bone-tendon junction of the greater tuberosity and passed through holes in the humeral implant. An additional suture can be passed around the collar of the implant and passed through the lesser tuberosity. Two additional sutures from the greater tuberosity are anchored through drill holes in the humeral shaft to provide vertical fixation. Vertical sutures are tied after the horizontal sutures to prevent distal position of the tuberosity. Bone graft from the removed humeral head is commonly used to improve the healing environment between the tuberosity, implant, and humeral shaft (**Box 2**).

Box 2
Reverse total shoulder arthroplasty (RTSA) key points

1. Functional outcome is improved with healing of the tuberosities in 3-part or 4-part proximal humerus fractures treated with RTSA

2. Press-fit or cemented stem is acceptable; however, minimal data are available to support either as the gold standard

3. Grafting of the tuberosities may improve healing rates

SUMMARY/DISCUSSION

Proximal humerus fracture treatment in patients with osteoporotic bone remains a challenge in terms of when and how to operate. Complications remain high with operative fixation of fractures. RTSA for severe fractures in elderly individuals is outpacing hemiarthroplasty in the United States. The treating surgeon should have several adjuncts to fixation available for these cases, as they can be somewhat unpredictable, and fixation can be tenuous.

REFERENCES

1. Court-Brown CM, Garg A, McQueen MM. The epidemiology of proximal humeral fractures. Acta Orthop Scand 2001;72(4):365–71.

2. Bell JE, Leung BC, Spratt KF, et al. Trends and variation in incidence, surgical treatment, and repeat surgery of proximal humeral fractures in the elderly. J Bone Joint Surg Am 2011;93(2):121–31.

3. Lee SH, Dargent-Molina P, Breart G, EPIDOS Group. Epidemiologie de l'Osteoporose Study. Risk factors for fractures of the proximal humerus: results from the EPIDOS prospective study. J Bone Miner Res 2002;17(5):817–25.

4. Rangan A, Handoll H, Brealey S, et al. Surgical vs nonsurgical treatment of adults with displaced

fractures of the proximal humerus: the PROFHER randomized clinical trial. JAMA 2015;313(10):1037–47.

5. Gardner MJ, Boraiah S, Helfet DL, et al. The anterolateral acromial approach for fractures of the proximal humerus. J Orthop Trauma 2008;22(2):132–7.

6. Seebeck J, Goldhahn J, Stadele H, et al. Effect of cortical thickness and cancellous bone density on the holding strength of internal fixator screws. J Orthop Res 2004;22(6):1237–42.

7. Seide K, Triebe J, Faschingbauer M, et al. Locked vs. unlocked plate osteosynthesis of the proximal humerus—a biomechanical study. Clin Biomech (Bristol, Avon) 2007;22(2):176–82.

8. Sproul RC, Iyengar JJ, Devcic Z, et al. A systematic review of locking plate fixation of proximal humerus fractures. Injury 2011;42(4):408–13.

9. Owsley KC, Gorczyca JT. Fracture displacement and screw cutout after open reduction and locked plate fixation of proximal humeral fractures [corrected]. J Bone Joint Surg Am 2008;90(2):233–40.

10. Jost B, Spross C, Grehn H, et al. Locking plate fixation of fractures of the proximal humerus: analysis of complications, revision strategies and outcome. J Shoulder Elbow Surg 2013;22(4):542–9.

11. Sudkamp N, Bayer J, Hepp P, et al. Open reduction and internal fixation of proximal humeral fractures with use of the locking proximal humerus plate. Results of a prospective, multicenter, observational study. J Bone Joint Surg Am 2009;91(6):1320–8.

12. Solberg BD, Moon CN, Franco DP, et al. Surgical treatment of three and four-part proximal humeral fractures. J Bone Joint Surg Am 2009;91(7):1689–97.

13. Schnetzke M, Bockmeyer J, Porschke F, et al. Quality of reduction influences outcome after locked-plate fixation of proximal humeral type-C fractures. J Bone Joint Surg Am 2016;98(21):1777–85.

14. Gardner MJ, Weil Y, Barker JU, et al. The importance of medial support in locked plating of proximal humerus fractures. J Orthop Trauma 2007; 21(3):185–91.

15. Bai L, Fu Z, An S, et al. Effect of calcar screw use in surgical neck fractures of the proximal humerus with unstable medial support: a biomechanical study. J Orthop Trauma 2014;28(8):452–7.

16. Katthagen JC, Schwarze M, Meyer-Kobbe J, et al. Biomechanical effects of calcar screws and bone block augmentation on medial support in locked plating of proximal humeral fractures. Clin Biomech (Bristol, Avon) 2014;29(7):735–41.

17. Ponce BA, Thompson KJ, Raghava P, et al. The role of medial comminution and calcar restoration in varus collapse of proximal humeral fractures treated with locking plates. J Bone Joint Surg Am 2013;95(16):e113(1-7).

18. Mehta S, Chin M, Sanville J, et al. Calcar screw position in proximal humerus fracture fixation: don't miss high! Injury 2018;49(3):624–9.

19. Padegimas EM, Zmistowski B, Lawrence C, et al. Defining optimal calcar screw positioning in proximal humerus fracture fixation. J Shoulder Elbow Surg 2017;26(11):1931–7.

20. Voigt C, Hurschler C, Rechi L, et al. Additive fiber-cerclages in proximal humeral fractures stabilized by locking plates: no effect on fracture stabilization and rotator cuff function in human shoulder specimens. Acta Orthop 2009;80(4):465–71.

21. Arvesen JE, Gill SW, Sinatra PM, et al. Biomechanical contribution of tension-reducing rotator cuff sutures in 3-part proximal humerus fractures. J Orthop Trauma 2016;30(8):e262–6.

22. Sinatra PM, Jernick ML, Bledsoe G, et al. No contribution of tension-reducing rotator cuff sutures on locking plate fixation in a 2-part proximal humerus fracture model. J Orthop Trauma 2014;28(8): 458–63.

23. Tingart MJ, Apreleva M, von Stechow D, et al. The cortical thickness of the proximal humeral diaphysis predicts bone mineral density of the proximal humerus. J Bone Joint Surg Br 2003;85(4):611–7.

24. Hepp P, Theopold J, Osterhoff G, et al. Bone quality measured by the radiogrammetric parameter "cortical index" and reoperations after locking plate osteosynthesis in patients sustaining proximal humerus fractures. Arch Orthop Trauma Surg 2009; 129(9):1251–9.

25. Bloom RA. A comparative estimation of the combined cortical thickness of various bone sites. Skeletal Radiol 1980;5(3):167–70.

26. Krappinger D, Roth T, Gschwentner M, et al. Preoperative assessment of the cancellous bone mineral density of the proximal humerus using CT data. Skeletal Radiol 2012;41(3):299–304.

27. Varga P, Grunwald L, Windolf M. The prediction of cyclic proximal humerus fracture fixation failure by various bone density measures. J Orthop Res 2018. https://doi.org/10.1002/jor.23879.

28. Walch G, Badet R, Nove-Josserand L, et al. Nonunions of the surgical neck of the humerus: surgical treatment with an intramedullary bone peg, internal fixation, and cancellous bone grafting. J Shoulder Elbow Surg 1996;5(3):161–8.

29. Gardner MJ, Boraiah S, Helfet DL, et al. Indirect medial reduction and strut support of proximal humerus fractures using an endosteal implant. J Orthop Trauma 2008;22(3):195–200.

30. Bae JH, Oh JK, Chon CS, et al. The biomechanical performance of locking plate fixation with intramedullary fibular strut graft augmentation in the treatment of unstable fractures of the proximal humerus. J Bone Joint Surg Br 2011;93(7):937–41.

31. Chow RM, Begum F, Beaupre LA, et al. Proximal humeral fracture fixation: locking plate construct +/− intramedullary fibular allograft. J Shoulder Elbow Surg 2012;21(7):894–901.

32. Mathison C, Chaudhary R, Beaupre L, et al. Biomechanical analysis of proximal humeral fixation using locking plate fixation with an intramedullary fibular allograft. Clin Biomech (Bristol, Avon) 2010;25(7): 642–6.

33. Ricchetti ET, Warrender WJ, Abboud JA. Use of locking plates in the treatment of proximal humerus fractures. J Shoulder Elbow Surg 2010;19(2 Suppl):66–75.

34. Kwon BK, Goertzen DJ, O'Brien PJ, et al. Biomechanical evaluation of proximal humeral fracture fixation supplemented with calcium phosphate cement. J Bone Joint Surg Am 2002;84-A(6): 951–61.

35. Egol KA, Sugi MT, Ong CC, et al. Fracture site augmentation with calcium phosphate cement reduces screw penetration after open reduction-internal fixation of proximal humeral fractures. J Shoulder Elbow Surg 2012;21(6):741–8.

36. Neer CS 2nd. Displaced proximal humeral fractures. I. Classification and evaluation. J Bone Joint Surg Am 1970;52(6):1077–89.

37. Neer CS 2nd. Displaced proximal humeral fractures. II. Treatment of three-part and four-part displacement. J Bone Joint Surg Am 1970;52(6): 1090–103.

38. Rajaee SS, Yalamanchili D, Noori N, et al. Increasing use of reverse total shoulder arthroplasty for proximal humerus fractures in elderly patients. Orthopedics 2017;40(6):e982–9.

39. Shukla DR, McAnany S, Kim J, et al. Hemiarthroplasty versus reverse shoulder arthroplasty for treatment of proximal humeral fractures: a meta-analysis. J Shoulder Elbow Surg 2016;25(2): 330–40.

40. Ferrel JR, Trinh TQ, Fischer RA. Reverse total shoulder arthroplasty versus hemiarthroplasty for proximal humeral fractures: a systematic review. J Orthop Trauma 2015;29(1):60–8.

41. Ladermann A, Walch G, Lubbeke A, et al. Influence of arm lengthening in reverse shoulder arthroplasty. J Shoulder Elbow Surg 2012;21(3):336–41.

42. Murachovsky J, Ikemoto RY, Nascimento LG, et al. Pectoralis major tendon reference (PMT): a new method for accurate restoration of humeral length with hemiarthroplasty for fracture. J Shoulder Elbow Surg 2006;15(6):675–8.

43. Ladermann A, Williams MD, Melis B, et al. Objective evaluation of lengthening in reverse shoulder arthroplasty. J Shoulder Elbow Surg 2009;18(4): 588–95.

44. Formaini NT, Everding NG, Levy JC, et al. Tuberosity healing after reverse shoulder arthroplasty for acute proximal humerus fractures: the "black and tan" technique. J Shoulder Elbow Surg 2015; 24(11):e299–306.

45. Chun YM, Kim DS, Lee DH, et al. Reverse shoulder arthroplasty for four-part proximal humerus fracture in elderly patients: can a healed tuberosity improve the functional outcomes? J Shoulder Elbow Surg 2017;26(7):1216–21.

46. Anakwenze OA, Zoller S, Ahmad CS, et al. Reverse shoulder arthroplasty for acute proximal humerus fractures: a systematic review. J Shoulder Elbow Surg 2014;23(4):e73–80.

47. Gallinet D, Adam A, Gasse N, et al. Improvement in shoulder rotation in complex shoulder fractures treated by reverse shoulder arthroplasty. J Shoulder Elbow Surg 2013;22(1):38–44.

48. Knierzinger D, Heinrichs CH, Hengg C, et al. Biomechanical evaluation of cable and suture cerclages for tuberosity reattachment in a 4-part proximal humeral fracture model treated with reverse shoulder arthroplasty. J Shoulder Elbow Surg 2018. https://doi.org/10.1016/j.jse.2018.04.003.

49. Uzer G, Yildiz F, Batar S, et al. Does grafting of the tuberosities improve the functional outcomes of proximal humeral fractures treated with reverse shoulder arthroplasty? J Shoulder Elbow Surg 2017;26(1):36–41.

50. Levy JC, Badman B. Reverse shoulder prosthesis for acute four-part fracture: tuberosity fixation using a horseshoe graft. J Orthop Trauma 2011; 25(5):318–24.

Surgical Considerations in Managing Osteoporosis, Osteopenia, and Vitamin D Deficiency During Arthroscopic Rotator Cuff Repair

Vahid Entezari, MD, MMSc[a],*, Mark Lazarus, MD[b,1]

KEYWORDS

• Rotator cuff tear • Rotator cuff repair • Bone quality • Osteopenia • Osteoporosis

---

KEY POINTS

• A patient with osteopenia and osteoporosis presents a difficult challenge for the surgeon contemplating arthroscopic rotator cuff repair.
• Deficiencies in bone mineralization have a profound effect on the greater tuberosity and thus can negatively impact rotator cuff repair healing.
• A thorough preoperative evaluation may reveal such a history so that an appropriate preoperative plan can be created.
• Several technical considerations exist that can help a surgeon achieve successful rotator cuff healing even in cases of severe greater tuberosity osseous deficiency.

INTRODUCTION

Rotator cuff tear (RCT) is a common cause of shoulder pain and dysfunction in adult patients.[1] In the United States alone, rotator cuff pathologies generate 4.5 million office visits and 250,000 surgeries per year.[2] The prevalence of RCT is 21% to 34% in asymptomatic subjects and it closely correlates with patient age.[3–6] The natural history of asymptomatic RCTs shows that after more than 2 years of follow-up, 39% of RCTs progress in size and 50% of patients with tear progression develop pain and dysfunction.[7,8] Chronic RCTs result in fatty infiltration and muscle atrophy, which negatively impacts the outcome of their treatment.[9,10] Although some tears, particularly in elderly patients, can be treated nonoperatively, the best outcome is achieved with operative treatment followed by tendon healing.[11] Rotator cuff tendon frequently heals after repair in younger patients with small size tear but re-tear rate is reported to be as high as 34% to 95%.[12,13] Risk factors for tendon re-tear are initial tear size,[14] tendon retraction,[15] fatty infiltration,[16] repair technique and patients' advanced age,[17] bone quality,[18] comorbidity,[19] and smoking status.[20] Among these factors, bone quality has received less attention, and the goal of this article was to review the role of osteoporosis, osteopenia, and vitamin D deficiency in rotator cuff repair and provide practical tips to manage poor bone quality during arthroscopic rotator cuff repair.

Disclosure Statement: The authors have nothing to disclose.
[a] Department of Orthopaedic Surgery, Orthopaedic & Rheumatologic Institute, Cleveland Clinic, 9500 Euclid Avenue, A40, Cleveland, OH 44195, USA; [b] Department of Orthopaedic Surgery, The Rothman Institute-Thomas Jefferson University, Philadelphia, PA, USA
[1] Present address: 9500 Euclid Avenue, A40, Cleveland, OH 44195.
* Corresponding author.
E-mail address: entezav@ccf.org

BONE QUALITY AND ROTATOR CUFF REPAIR

Osteoporosis and Osteopenia

Osteoporosis is a chronic and progressive disease characterized by low bone density and microstructural deterioration in the skeleton commonly affecting postmenopausal women.[21] According to the World Health Organization's definition, bone mineral density (BMD) between 1.0 and 2.5 standard deviations (SDs) below the mean for young adult women is defined as osteopenia and more than 2.5 SDs is defined as osteoporosis.[22] In the United States alone, there are 18 million patients with osteopenia and 10 million patients with osteoporosis.[23] Based on 2005 estimates, osteoporosis resulted in more than 2 million incidents of fractures and $17 billion in direct medical costs.[24] The lifetime risk of fragility fracture for a 50-year-old patient is 17% for women and 6% for men. The etiology of low BMD is classified as primary, commonly affecting postmenopausal women, or secondary, caused by medications (eg, glucocorticoids, anticonvulsant therapy) or conditions such as endocrine abnormalities (eg, hypogonadism, hyperthyroidism) or malnutrition (eg, low calcium and vitamin D or alcohol abuse).[23]

Proximal Humerus Bone Quality

The bone quality of the proximal humerus has been studied extensively in the literature, including its effects on the risk of proximal humerus fracture and fixation strength of arthroplasty and arthroscopic implants. The failure rate of the rotator cuff repair has been reported as high as 68% and the bone quality of the greater tuberosity is thought to be one of the factors affecting the repair integrity.[25] Although the location of the tear, tendon retraction, and tissue quality can influence whether the repair can be achieved, the surgeon still controls the location, size and type of anchors, and the repair construct, and, therefore, it is key to understand how bone quality affects incidence of RCT and failure after repair.

The BMD of the proximal humerus is highly variable between subjects and it diminishes as patients age, with the most pronounced deterioration observed in women older than 70 years.[26,27] Doetsch and colleagues[28] performed dual-energy X-ray absorptimetry (DEXA) scan on the dominant shoulder in 80 healthy subjects and reported that shoulder BMD was significantly lower than hip BMD and the difference had a positive correlation with patient's body mass index. This suggests that the non–weight-bearing nature of the proximal

humerus makes it more prone to disuse osteopenia and the standard means to assess patients' bone quality can underestimate proximal humerus BMD especially in obese patients. The 2-dimensional nature of the DEXA images limits its ability to assess the special distribution of the bone and bone microstructure, which is highly relevant to rotator cuff disease and repair. Tingart and colleagues[25] studied the 3-dimensional (3D) distribution of the bone in the proximal humerus using peripheral quantitative computed tomography (CT) and demonstrated that the intertubercular area has the highest density of bone in the proximal humerus. Using CT imaging also has the advantage of evaluating both the cortical and trabecular bone, which may have clinical significance. For example, Kirchhoff and colleagues[29] performed high-resolution quantitative CT imaging on 36 cadaveric shoulders with a mean age of 75 years. They showed that the cancellous bone of the greater and lesser tuberosities has decreasing bone quality with deeper slices, which implies that placement of suture anchors into deeper cancellous regions of the humeral head will not result in increased stability.

Several studies have reported an association between RCT and reduced BMD of the greater tuberosity.[30–34] Galatz and colleagues[35] studied the effect of delayed repair of the supraspinatus tendon tear in 60 rats with transected tendon and found that the delayed repair group not only had worse viscoelastic properties tendon repair but also showed decreased greater tuberosity bone density. Waldorff and colleagues[31] measured greater tuberosity bone density using digital radiographs and showed greater tuberosity osteopenia in patients with full-thickness and partial-thickness RCTs as compared with the control group and suggested bony changes might predate rotator cuff disease. As indicated before, studies that used 3D CT analysis report more granular data on regional variation of bone density and are more clinically relevant. Meyer and colleagues[30] performed micro-CT analysis of the proximal humerus on 7 pairs of cadaveric shoulders and showed the ones with full-thickness RCT had greater than 50% reduction in their greater tuberosity cancellous bone density compared with the shoulders with no RCT, whereas bone density was better preserved below the articular surface. Oh and colleagues[32] obtained bilateral CT scan and measured volumetric BMD on a cohort of 65 patients who underwent arthroscopic repair for unilateral RCT. They found that BMD of the greater tuberosity was significantly lower in the shoulder with RCT and bone density within the greater tuberosity was highest in the posterolateral followed by anterolateral region. The investigators warn against relying on medial row fixation especially in elderly female patients as this area had the lowest BMD in their cohort. Evidence from the finite element analysis of the strain distribution over the humeral head reveals that rotator cuff stress over the greater tuberosity does not penetrate deep into the cancellous bone[36] and high grade RCTs with retraction can rapidly affect mineralization of the subcortical bone in this region.[37]

Several studies assessed the relationship between the bone quality of the greater tuberosity and suture anchor pullout strength.[38,39] Unfortunately, studies on this topic have variable imaging and mechanical testing protocols, which makes it difficult to compare and contrast their findings. Barber and colleagues[38] attempted to correlate DEXA-based BMD of the greater tuberosity with the pullout strength of the suture anchor in a cadaveric model. They found greater pullout strength in the posterior greater tuberosity but failed to show a difference in BMD between anterior and posterior tuberosity region. These results have been criticized mainly due to an inherent limitation of the DEXA imaging in assessing the bone microstructure. Tingart and colleagues[39] evaluated suture pullout strength in 17 cadaveric humeri and correlated it with the CT-based BMD measurements. Although their CT images had low resolution with pixel size of only 0.59 mm, they found positive correlation between greater tuberosity BMD and suture anchor pullout strength. Based on their data within the proximal tuberosity area, load to failure of suture anchors in the anterior and middle regions was 62% higher than the posterior region ($P<.01$).

In summary, the bone quality of the greater tuberosity deteriorates with aging, especially in female patients (Box 1). Patients with RCTs show diminished BMD of the greater tuberosity, which affects the pullout strength of the suture anchors used during the repair. There is convincing evidence that subchondral and cortical bone density is better preserved than cancellous bone, and surgeons should prohibit aggressive decortications of the tuberosity region. Also studying the cancellous bone microarchitecture of the greater tuberosity shows that deeper regions of the greater tuberosity have worse properties and deep insertion of suture anchors into the humeral head should be avoided. Although the intertubercular region has the highest BMD in the proximal humerus,

there is no consensus on where suture anchors should be placed within the greater tuberosity mainly due to variability in imaging and biomechanical protocols of studies in the literature.

Vitamin D Deficiency

Vitamin D maintains calcium and phosphate homeostasis in the body. When sunlight hits the skin, ultraviolet radiation transforms 7-dehydrocholesterol to pre-vitamin D3, which then is metabolized in the liver to 25-hydroxyvitamin D3 (calcifediol).[40] Finally, calcifediol is metabolized to 1,25-dihydroxivitamin D3 or the active form of vitamin D in the kidneys. Vitamin D and its precursors promote absorption of calcium and regulate circulating levels of calcium and phosphate for normal bone mineralization. Also, vitamin D plays an important role in decreasing inflammatory response through downregulating proinflammatory cytokines, such as tumor necrosis factor alpha and interleukin-6,[41] promoting protein synthesis and skeletal muscle growth[42,43] and also is implicated in fracture healing.[44,45]

Box 1
Proximal humerus osteopenia and osteoporosis

- Proximal humerus bone mineral density diminishes with aging
- Female patients, especially those older than 70 years, are high risk for greater tuberosity osteopenia
- Intertubercular region has the highest bone mineral density in the humeral head
- Distribution of bone density within the greater tuberosity has high variability
- Cortical density remains less affected than cancellous bone and decortication of the tuberosity should be minimized in elderly and patients with poor bone quality
- High-resolution 3-dimensional computed tomography data suggest that anterior and intermediate regions might have higher cancellous bone density compared to the posterior region
- The microarchitecture of the cancellous bone deteriorates in deeper regions, making the cortical and superficial trabecular bone the best area to achieve fixation
- Rotator cuff tear results in diminished bone mineral density of the greater tuberosity, most probably due to a combination of disuse and lack of rotator cuff stress over the tuberosity

Vitamin D deficiency is defined as 25-hydroxyvitamin D level ≤20 ng/mL (50 nmol/L).[46] It is estimated that 1 billion people in the world are suffering from vitamin D deficiency.[47] Prevalence of vitamin D deficiency is 36% to 47% in general population in the US and European adults,[48] and 58% to 76% in patients with hip fracture.[49,50] Vitamin D deficiency is associated with advanced age,[51,52] nonwhite race, low education level, obesity, less milk consumption,[48] diabetes,[53] cardiovascular disease,[54] and cancer.[55] Vitamin D deficiency has also been linked to low physical performance[56] and elderly falls.[57] Supplementation of vitamin D and calcium has shown to slow postmenopausal bone loss,[58] reduce risk of osteoporotic fracture,[59] and potentially reduce tendency to fall in elderly patients.[60]

The link between vitamin D and rotator cuff muscle fatty infiltration was first reported by Oh and colleagues.[61] In their cross-sectional study, patients with shoulder symptoms who underwent MRI were categorized into patients with full-thickness RCTs (n = 228) and patients without full-thickness RCTs (n = 138), and their serum 25-hydroxyvitamin D3 level and isokinetic muscle torque were measured. They found that higher fatty infiltration was correlated with advanced age, female gender, full-thickness tear, size and retraction of the tear, lower abduction and external rotation torque, and lower vitamin D level. In their multivariate regression analysis, lower level of vitamin D was an independent predictor of fatty infiltration in supraspinatus and infraspinatus muscles ($P = .001$) and bilateral isokinetic muscle torque ($P<.001$). There was a dose-effect relationship between muscle atrophy grade and level of vitamin D but it did not reach statistical significance.

The effect of vitamin D on tendon repair is another emerging area of study that has direct relevance to rotator cuff treatment. Native tendon-to-bone insertion has a complex anatomy with 4 distinct zones including tendon, unmineralized fibrocartilage, mineralized fibrocartilage, and bone. Each zone has unique histologic and biochemical make-up.[62] It has been shown that scar that is formed at the site of the tendon repair lacks this structural differentiation and is weaker than the original tendon.[42] Angeline and colleagues[63] showed that in a rat model of rotator cuff repair, vitamin D sufficient rats had greater load to failure and better organization of collagen fibers at the site of the repair. Ryu and colleagues[64] also evaluated the relationship between preoperative vitamin D level and severity of RCT and risk of re-tear in 91 consecutive patients who underwent rotator

cuff repair. They found no relationship between vitamin D level and preoperative tear size, retraction and degree of fatty infiltration, and postoperative repair integrity and functional outcome. One important limitation of this study was that 88% of these patients were vitamin D deficient and only 3 patients had sufficient levels of vitamin D. Overall, larger randomized control trials are needed to delineate the effect of vitamin D level on RCT and muscle fatty infiltration, and a possible role for vitamin D supplementation in rotator cuff repair.

Clinical Evaluation

Clinical evaluation of patients with RCTs should include obtaining a thorough history and physical examination. The surgeon should pay attention to presenting symptoms, their nature, duration, location, severity, and aggravating and alleviating factors. The hand dominance, occupation, level of physical activity, history of acute injury, and baseline pain and function of the arm should be obtained. Past medical history of diabetes, chronic inflammatory and endocrine disease, nutritional abnormalities, and any congenital disease that can affect bone quality should be reviewed. History of osteopenia, osteoporosis, generalized body aching, lack of mobility, tendency to fall, any fragility fracture, and treatments that can affect bone quality, including steroids, calcium, vitamin D, antiresorptive medications, and history of smoking and alcohol abuse, should be obtained. Physical examination should not only focus on delineating the severity of symptoms related to rotator cuff, but the surgeon should pay close attention to muscle atrophy from chronic RCT and kyphotic posture from diffuse osteoporotic vertebral collapse.

Imaging

Preoperative imaging for patients with RCTs commonly includes a set of plain radiographs and MRI, but may include a CT arthrogram or ultrasound evaluation. Plain radiographs are ordered to assess the osseous structure of the shoulder, presence of glenohumeral and acromioclavicular arthritis, and degree of humeral head migration. Generally, plain radiograph is not the most accurate modality to assess bone quality, but Tingart and colleagues[65] showed that cortical thickness of humeral shaft measured at 2 specific levels distal to the surgical neck is highly predictive of BMD of the proximal humerus measured by DEXA scan. For the patient who presents with a rotator cuff re-tear after prior repair, plain radiographs may reveal anchor loosening or pullout, which suggests humeral head osteopenia (Fig. 1). CT scan provides high-resolution 3D images of bony structures in the shoulder and allows for better appreciation of bone stock and focal and generalized bone loss. Many CT-based quantitative measurements have been developed to assess the BMD of the greater tuberosity and its microarchitecture, but most have only research application. MRI is the study of choice to assess the size and location of the tear and associated tendon retraction, fatty infiltration, and muscle atrophy. Other findings, such as size and location of the subchondral cysts, presence of humeral head cavitary lesions, or collapse of the humeral head, will give surgeons better appreciation of possible technical challenges they may face during the rotator cuff repair.

Treatment

Rotator cuff repair has high re-tear rate and the risk of failure increases with patients' advancing age[66] and larger tear size.[67] The quality of the proximal humerus bone also deteriorates with aging and is more pronounced in patients who have RCT. Djurasovic and colleagues[68] reviewed 80 cases of failed rotator cuff repair and showed 10% of them had anchor migration or loosening. Also, RCT chronicity usually coincides with advanced age, larger tear size, and poor soft tissue and bone quality that can complicate a surgeon's ability to mobilize, reduce, and successfully repair the tendon back to its native footprint. The open versus arthroscopic rotator cuff repair debate continues, as many preliminary studies showed a slight advantage in healing rate of mini-open over arthroscopic repair techniques. A recent randomized controlled trial by Carr and colleagues[69] showed no difference in success rate of mini-open versus arthroscopic rotator cuff repair for all ages and tear sizes.

Multiple systematic reviews also found no difference between the outcomes of these 2 techniques.[70] Arthroscopic rotator cuff repair continues to gain popularity, while experience with open rotator cuff repair is dwindling among the new generation of surgeons. As emphasized by Denard and Burkhart,[71] there are general technical and biomechanical principles that should be followed in handling of the soft tissue and bone to improve the success rate of rotator cuff repair in this patient population (Box 2). This

> **Box 2**
> **Technical pearls for repairing rotator cuff tear in patients with poor bone quality**
>
> - Visualize, mobilize, and recognize tear pattern
> - Minimize tuberosity shaving to preserve as much bone as possible
> - Identify areas with the large cystic changes on the MRI and CT scan, and, if possible, avoid putting anchors in those areas
> - Mobilize the rotator cuff to reduce the tension off the repair
> - If dealing with a chronically retracted rotator cuff tear, consider single row partial repair and even advancing the medial row anchors onto the humeral head to reduce the tension on the repair
> - Avoid fully punching anchor holes if bone quality is poor; start the holes with the punch and let the anchor impact the cancellous bone within the head
> - If the anchor pulls out or does not achieve sufficient fixation, attempt removal and upsizing
> - Try to put anterior anchors closer to the bicipital groove where the bone quality is better
> - If possible, increase the number of anchors to distribute tension across multiple anchors
> - Place anchors at 90° angles to the cortical surface, as there is empirical evidence that perpendicular insertion of threaded anchors will increase the pullout strength compared with 45°
> - Use suture tapes that have the hypothetical advantage of distributing the force over the larger area
> - Use anchorless transosseous technique, which reduces the area required for passage of sutures relative to the size of the footprint and rigidity of the overall construct is not dependent on anchor-bone fixation

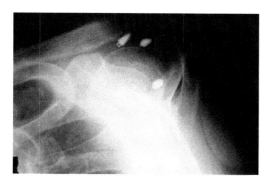

Fig. 1. Loose metal anchors associated with rotator cuff repair failure in a patient with known history of osteoporosis.

section focuses on the technical pearls and biomechanical principals that are most relevant to arthroscopic rotator cuff repair.

Visualize the entire rotator cuff tear, mobilize the torn tendons, and recognize the tear size, location, pattern, retraction, and associated pathologies

Appropriate treatment of any RCT starts with a good diagnostic evaluation, which begins with an intra-articular evaluation of the long head of the biceps tendon, labrum, capsule, and the cartilage, and then focuses on identifying the size, location, pattern, retraction, and mobility of the torn tendons. The "interval slide" technique has been advocated to detach the anterior retracted edge of the supraspinatus tendon from underlying capsule, coracohumeral ligament, and interval tissue from lateral to medial under direct visualization.[72] This concept has also been applied to developing the interval between supraspinatus and infraspinatus tendons to release adhesions between the retracted cuff and spine of the scapula.[73] Thorough debridement of the scar, adhesions, and remnants of the tendon covering the tuberosity and freshening of the tendon edges will improve visualization and help with recognizing the tear pattern and intraoperative planning for the repair. There have been multiple studies that show the addition of formal subacromial decompression to rotator cuff repair does not change patients' re-tear rate and patient-reported outcome.[74,75] As was discussed earlier, surgeons should avoid aggressive shaving and decortications of the tuberosity, because in patients with poor bone quality, cortical bone might be the only reliable fixation point for the rotator cuff repair.

Increase the number of fixation points

Increasing the number of fixation points reduces the stress concentration over the anchor-bone and suture-tendon interface. The limiting factor in the number of anchors per tear is the size of the footprint. Kawakami and colleagues[76] showed in a polyurethane and porcine model that minimum distance between the anchors without decreasing the pullout strength was 6 mm, which is smaller than 10-mm distance that was previously established and this did not change with the specimen's bone quality. Despite these cadaveric data, the surgeon should balance the number of anchors with the size of the RCT, footprint area, and intraoperative assessment of the bone quality.

Use appropriate suture configuration to maximize soft tissue grip and footprint compression

The most common suture anchor configurations used in rotator cuff repair are single row (SR), double row (DR), and transosseous equivalent (TOE). The SR repair includes passage of 1 row of sutures through the cuff, and DR repair includes addition of a lateral row of anchors in an attempt to recreate the native rotator cuff footprint attachment.[77] The TOE is technically a DR suture configuration in which 1 limb from each medial anchor is crossed and included in a lateral distal row of anchors to compress the tendon over the footprint and optimize tendon-to-tuberosity contact area.[78] There are limited clinical data to compare SR, DR, and TOE repair techniques. Biomechanical data suggest that DR repair might be slightly superior to SR repair in restoring the strength and minimizing the gap formation at the repair site.[79] A systematic review by Chen and colleagues[80] revealed that DR repair is more beneficial in large-size tears. On the contrary, another systematic review found that patient-reported outcomes were not different between the SR and DR repair. The advantage of TOE over DR is tendon-bone compression and higher contact area. McCormick and colleagues compared results of SR, DR, and TOE in 63 patients with a torn supraspinatus and minimum 2-year follow-up, and their MRI based re-tear rates were 22%, 18%, and 11%, respectively, but their diffidence did not reach statistical significance. Mihata and colleagues[81] also reported their minimum 2-year results of SR, DR, and TOE technique in 206 consecutive patients and reported re-tear rate of 10.8%, 26.1%, and 4.7%, respectively.

From a bone-quality standpoint, all 3 suture configurations rely on suture anchors for fixation. The advantage of SR technique is the speed and lower cost. The SR repair can be applied in patients in whom the rotator cuff could not be mobilized to cover the entire footprint. The DR and TOE repairs rely on more than 1 row of suture anchors and reduce the force concentrated on each anchor. The TOE repair has a few advantages over the DR, which include tendon coverage of the greater tuberosity, compression over the footprint area, and transferring the lateral row to more distal aspect of the tuberosity with potentially better bone quality.

Use larger suture anchors

Using larger suture anchors with minimum punching will improve the odds of achieving sufficient anchor fixation.

There might be a role for metal anchors
Using metal anchors may also increase the chance of successful fixation. Tingart and colleagues[82] compared the pullout strength of metal and biodegradable suture anchors after cyclic loading and found metallic anchors had significantly higher pullout strength than biodegradable anchors. Despite the superior biomechanical performance, Milano and colleagues[83] in a randomized controlled trial showed similar patient-reported outcome at minimum 2 years in 110 patients who underwent rotator cuff repair with metallic and biodegradable suture anchors.

Insert anchors perpendicular to the tuberosity surface
The theory of "deadman angle" was introduced by Burkhart[84] in 1995 based on mathematical calculations and suggested that reducing the angle between suture anchor and the rotator cuff tendon will result in higher pullout strength. Strauss and colleagues[85] tested the hypothesis in a cadaveric model with varying angle of anchor insertion from 45 to 90° and compared number of cycles leading to 3-mm gap formation in the tendon. They found that complete failure happened at a significantly higher number of cycles when the anchor was inserted at 90° compared with 45° ($P<.005$). Therefore, perpendicular insertion of threaded anchors appears to increase the suture anchor pullout strength compared with 45°.[86]

Transosseous anchorless fixation technique
The advent of suture anchors helped with popularizing arthroscopic rotator cuff repair due to ease and speed of use and facilitating the instrumentation.[39] The design and material used in suture anchors has gone through a tremendous evolution and improved our ability to achieve better rotator cuff repair. Nonetheless, suture anchors rely heavily on the bone-anchor interface for providing stable fixation while biologic healing occurs. Many studies have shown that the anchor-bone interface is the "weak link" in the suture anchor rotator cuff repair construct. Loosening of a suture anchor within the greater tuberosity can result in the loss of fixation of the rotator cuff repair and can lead to re-tear and large cavitary lesions due to micromotion of the loose implant (**Fig. 2**). The arthroscopic transosseous anchorless repair is a technique that, instead of relying on suture anchors, achieves fixation via sutures and tapes passed through bone tunnels within the humeral head (**Fig. 3**). Also, in patients with very poor bone

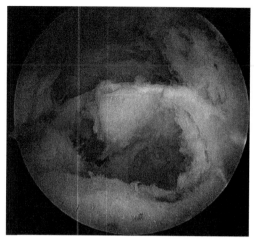

Fig. 2. Arthroscopic image of a loose suture anchor in a patient with poor bone quality, which resulted in a large bone defect within the greater tuberosity.

quality, support plugs are used to support transosseous canals (**Fig. 4**). This technique is very attractive because it does not use any suture anchors and results in substantial cost saving. Black and colleagues[87] showed that the cost per case was significantly higher with TOE than anchorless, approaching $800 in massive cuff tear. Although average case duration was similar between TOE and anchorless technique (98 vs 99 minutes), the anchorless technique had a steeper learning curve with suture management and was more sensitive to increasing tear size.

Bone grafting and cement augmentation
One of the methods to address poor bone quality in rotator cuff repair is to bone graft or use

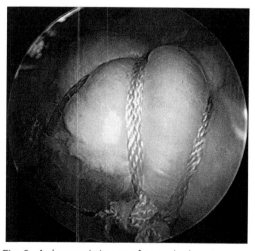

Fig. 3. Arthroscopic image of an anchorless, transosseous suture repair with uniform compression of the rotator cuff over the footprint area without reliance to suture anchors.

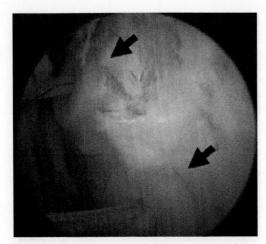

Fig. 4. Arthroscopic image of plugs (*arrows*) used in an anchorless, transosseous suture repair supporting tunnels in a patient with poor bone quality.

cement augmentation to fill the void created by osteoporotic bone resorption or large cystic changes within the subchondral plate. Structural bone grafting, especially in the arthroscopic setting, is technically challenging and would not provide immediate improvement in the fixation strength. This has encouraged researchers to look for other means of augmentation at the time of repair. Structural augmentation of the poor bone quality can be achieved through introduction of an injectable material that is able to fill the void and interdigitate with surrounding bone. Oshtory and colleagues[82] reported 29% increase in pullout strength of suture anchors augmented with tricalcium phosphate. Giori and colleagues[88] showed suture anchors that were placed in polymethylmethacrylate had 71% increased maximum load compared with anchors placed in bone. Aziz and colleagues[89] reported 62% higher pullout strength of suture anchors with the cement injected through the anchor into the humeral head compared with conventional anchors in a cadaveric human model. Despite these promising results, more studies are needed to establish the impact of augmentation techniques on in vivo biomechanical properties and long-term performance of the repair. Also, there are concerns regarding extra cost, extravasation of the augmentation material into the joint, its effect on the bone-tendon healing, and the potential added difficulty of future surgeries.

Convert to open rotator cuff repair
Although the specific topic of this review is the consideration of poor bone quality in arthroscopic rotator cuff repair, when all else fails, a solution is to convert to an open repair. The

cortical thickness of the proximal humerus is better the more distal from the greater tuberosity that fixation is attempted. Creating arthroscopic transosseous tunnels distal in the lateral humeral cortex is technically difficult, but relatively easy when done open. In general, even in the severely osteoporotic patient, successful osseous fixation can be accomplished by transosseous fixation with the lateral bone tunnel created distal on the lateral humeral cortex.

SUMMARY

A patient with osteopenia and osteoporosis presents a difficult challenge for the surgeon contemplating arthroscopic rotator cuff repair. Deficiencies in bone mineralization have a profound effect on the BMD of the greater tuberosity and thus can negatively impact rotator cuff repair healing. A thorough preoperative evaluation may reveal such a history so that an appropriate preoperative plan can be created. Several technical considerations exist that can help surgeons achieve successful rotator cuff healing even in cases of severe greater tuberosity osseous deficiency.

REFERENCES

1. Urwin M, Symmons D, Allison T, et al. Estimating the burden of musculoskeletal disorders in the community: the comparative prevalence of symptoms at different anatomical sites, and the relation to social deprivation. Ann Rheum Dis 1998;57: 649–55.
2. Oh LS, Wolf BR, Hall MP, et al. Indications for rotator cuff repair: a systematic review. Clin Orthop Relat Res 2007;455:52–63.
3. Yamaguchi K, Ditsios K, Middleton WD, et al. The demographic and morphological features of rotator cuff disease. A comparison of asymptomatic and symptomatic shoulders. J Bone Joint Surg Am 2006;88:1699–704.
4. Minagawa A, Koga H, Uhara H, et al. Age-related prevalence of dermoscopic patterns in acquired melanocytic nevus on acral volar skin. JAMA Dermatol 2013;149:989–90.
5. Sher JS, Uribe JW, Posada A, et al. Abnormal findings on magnetic resonance images of asymptomatic shoulders. J Bone Joint Surg Am 1995;77:10–5.
6. Sayampanathan AA, Andrew TH. Systematic review on risk factors of rotator cuff tears. J Orthop Surg (Hong Kong) 2017;25. 2309499016684318.
7. Keener JD, Galatz LM, Teefey SA, et al. A prospective evaluation of survivorship of asymptomatic degenerative rotator cuff tears. J Bone Joint Surg Am 2015;97:89–98.

8. Yamaguchi K, Tetro AM, Blam O, et al. Natural history of asymptomatic rotator cuff tears: a longitudinal analysis of asymptomatic tears detected sonographically. J Shoulder Elbow Surg 2001;10: 199–203.

9. Gladstone JN, Bishop JY, Lo IK, et al. Fatty infiltration and atrophy of the rotator cuff do not improve after rotator cuff repair and correlate with poor functional outcome. Am J Sports Med 2007;35: 719–28.

10. Kim HM, Dahiya N, Teefey SA, et al. Relationship of tear size and location to fatty degeneration of the rotator cuff. J Bone Joint Surg Am 2010;92:829–39.

11. Park JY, Lhee SH, Oh KS, et al. Clinical and ultrasonographic outcomes of arthroscopic suture bridge repair for massive rotator cuff tear. Arthroscopy 2013;29:280–9.

12. Galatz LM, Ball CM, Teefey SA, et al. The outcome and repair integrity of completely arthroscopically repaired large and massive rotator cuff tears. J Bone Joint Surg Am 2004;86-A:219–24.

13. Gerber C, Fuchs B, Hodler J. The results of repair of massive tears of the rotator cuff. J Bone Joint Surg Am 2000;82:505–15.

14. Gazielly DF, Gleyze P, Montagnon C. Functional and anatomical results after rotator cuff repair. Clin Orthop Relat Res 1994;(304):43–53.

15. Shin YK, Ryu KN, Park JS, et al. Predictive factors of retear in patients with repaired rotator cuff tear on shoulder MRI. AJR Am J Roentgenol 2018;210: 134–41.

16. Liem D, Lichtenberg S, Magosch P, et al. Magnetic resonance imaging of arthroscopic supraspinatus tendon repair. J Bone Joint Surg Am 2007;89: 1770–6.

17. Nho SJ, Brown BS, Lyman S, et al. Prospective analysis of arthroscopic rotator cuff repair: prognostic factors affecting clinical and ultrasound outcome. J Shoulder Elbow Surg 2009;18:13–20.

18. Chung SW, Oh JH, Gong HS, et al. Factors affecting rotator cuff healing after arthroscopic repair: osteoporosis as one of the independent risk factors. Am J Sports Med 2011;39:2099–107.

19. Abtahi AM, Granger EK, Tashjian RZ. Factors affecting healing after arthroscopic rotator cuff repair. World J Orthop 2015;6:211–20.

20. Neyton L, Godeneche A, Nove-Josserand L, et al. Arthroscopic suture-bridge repair for small to medium size supraspinatus tear: healing rate and retear pattern. Arthroscopy 2013;29:10–7.

21. Cooper C, Melton LJ 3rd. Epidemiology of osteoporosis. Trends Endocrinol Metab 1992;3:224–9.

22. Kanis JA, Melton LJ 3rd, Christiansen C, et al. The diagnosis of osteoporosis. J Bone Miner Res 1994;9:1137–41.

23. NIH consensus development panel on osteoporosis prevention, diagnosis, and therapy, March 7-

29, 2000: highlights of the conference. South Med J 2001;94:569–73.

24. Burge R, Dawson-Hughes B, Solomon DH, et al. Incidence and economic burden of osteoporosis-related fractures in the United States, 2005-2025. J Bone Miner Res 2007;22:465–75.

25. Tingart MJ, Bouxsein ML, Zurakowski D, et al. Three-dimensional distribution of bone density in the proximal humerus. Calcif Tissue Int 2003;73:531–6.

26. Park JY, Kim MH. Changes in bone mineral density of the proximal humerus in Koreans: suture anchor in rotator cuff repair. Orthopedics 2004;27:857–61.

27. Kirchhoff C, Braunstein V, Milz S, et al. Age and gender as determinants of the bone quality of the greater tuberosity: a HR-pQCT cadaver study. BMC Musculoskelet Disord 2012;13:221.

28. Doetsch AM, Faber J, Lynnerup N, et al. Bone mineral density measurement over the shoulder region. Calcif Tissue Int 2002;71:308–14.

29. Kirchhoff C, Kirchhoff S, Sprecher CM, et al. X-treme CT analysis of cancellous bone at the rotator cuff insertion in human individuals with osteoporosis: superficial versus deep quality. Arch Orthop Trauma Surg 2013;133:381–7.

30. Meyer DC, Fucentese SF, Koller B, et al. Association of osteopenia of the humeral head with full-thickness rotator cuff tears. J Shoulder Elbow Surg 2004;13:333–7.

31. Waldorff EI, Lindner J, Kijek TG, et al. Bone density of the greater tuberosity is decreased in rotator cuff disease with and without full-thickness tears. J Shoulder Elbow Surg 2011;20:904–8.

32. Oh JH, Song BW, Lee YS. Measurement of volumetric bone mineral density in proximal humerus using quantitative computed tomography in patients with unilateral rotator cuff tear. J Shoulder Elbow Surg 2014;23:993–1002.

33. Oh JH, Song BW, Kim SH, et al. The measurement of bone mineral density of bilateral proximal humeri using DXA in patients with unilateral rotator cuff tear. Osteoporos Int 2014;25:2639–48.

34. Kholinne E, Lee HJ, Kim SJ, et al. The relationship between age, rotator cuff integrity, and osseous microarchitecture of greater tuberosity: where should we put anchor? Acta Orthop Traumatol Turc 2018;52:22–6.

35. Galatz LM, Rothermich SY, Zaegel M, et al. Delayed repair of tendon to bone injuries leads to decreased biomechanical properties and bone loss. J Orthop Res 2005;23:1441–7.

36. Clavert P, Zerah M, Krier J, et al. Finite element analysis of the strain distribution in the humeral head tubercles during abduction: comparison of young and osteoporotic bone. Surg Radiol Anat 2006;28:581–7.

37. Clavert P, Bouchaib J, Sommaire C, et al. Does bone density of the greater tuberosity change in

patients over 70? Orthop Traumatol Surg Res 2014; 100:109–11.

38. Barber FA, Feder SM, Burkhart SS, et al. The relationship of suture anchor failure and bone density to proximal humerus location: a cadaveric study. Arthroscopy 1997;13:340–5.

39. Tingart MJ, Apreleva M, Zurakowski D, et al. Pullout strength of suture anchors used in rotator cuff repair. J Bone Joint Surg Am 2003;85-A: 2190–8.

40. Nossov S, Dines JS, Murrell GA, et al. Biologic augmentation of tendon-to-bone healing: scaffolds, mechanical load, vitamin D, and diabetes. Instr Course Lect 2014;63:451–62.

41. Guillot X, Semerano L, Saidenberg-Kermanac'h N, et al. Vitamin D and inflammation. Joint Bone Spine 2010;77:552–7.

42. Dougherty KA, Dilisio MF, Agrawal DK. Vitamin D and the immunomodulation of rotator cuff injury. J Inflamm Res 2016;9:123–31.

43. Birge SJ, Haddad JG. 25-hydroxycholecalciferol stimulation of muscle metabolism. J Clin Invest 1975;56:1100–7.

44. Doetsch AM, Faber J, Lynnerup N, et al. The effect of calcium and vitamin D3 supplementation on the healing of the proximal humerus fracture: a randomized placebo-controlled study. Calcif Tissue Int 2004;75:183–8.

45. Gorter EA, Hamdy NA, Appelman-Dijkstra NM, et al. The role of vitamin D in human fracture healing: a systematic review of the literature. Bone 2014;64:288–97.

46. Bischoff-Ferrari HA, Giovannucci E, Willett WC, et al. Estimation of optimal serum concentrations of 25-hydroxyvitamin D for multiple health outcomes. Am J Clin Nutr 2006;84:18–28.

47. Holick MF. Vitamin D deficiency. N Engl J Med 2007;357:266–81.

48. Forrest KY, Stuhldreher WL. Prevalence and correlates of vitamin D deficiency in US adults. Nutr Res 2011;31:48–54.

49. Ramason R, Selvaganapathi N, Ismail NH, et al. Prevalence of vitamin D deficiency in patients with hip fracture seen in an orthogeriatric service in sunny Singapore. Geriatr Orthop Surg Rehabil 2014;5:82–6.

50. Dhanwal DK, Sahoo S, Gautam VK, et al. Hip fracture patients in India have vitamin D deficiency and secondary hyperparathyroidism. Osteoporos Int 2013;24:553–7.

51. van der Wielen RP, Lowik MR, van den Berg H, et al. Serum vitamin D concentrations among elderly people in Europe. Lancet 1995;346:207–10.

52. Boucher BJ. The problems of vitamin D insufficiency in older people. Aging Dis 2012;3:313–29.

53. Boucher BJ. Vitamin D insufficiency and diabetes risks. Curr Drug Targets 2011;12:61–87.

54. Vaidya A, Forman JP. Vitamin D and vascular disease: the current and future status of vitamin D therapy in hypertension and kidney disease. Curr Hypertens Rep 2012;14:111–9.

55. Grant WB. Ecological studies of the UVB-vitamin D-cancer hypothesis. Anticancer Res 2012;32:223–36.

56. Annweiler C, Schott AM, Berrut G, et al. Vitamin D-related changes in physical performance: a systematic review. J Nutr Health Aging 2009;13:893–8.

57. Duval GT, Pare PY, Gautier J, et al. Vitamin D and the mechanisms, circumstances and consequences of falls in older adults: a case-control study. J Nutr Health Aging 2017;21:1307–13.

58. Ooms ME, Roos JC, Bezemer PD, et al. Prevention of bone loss by vitamin D supplementation in elderly women: a randomized double-blind trial. J Clin Endocrinol Metab 1995;80:1052–8.

59. Larsen ER, Mosekilde L, Foldspang A. Vitamin D and calcium supplementation prevents osteoporotic fractures in elderly community dwelling residents: a pragmatic population-based 3-year intervention study. J Bone Miner Res 2004;19: 370–8.

60. Annweiler C, Montero-Odasso M, Schott AM, et al. Fall prevention and vitamin D in the elderly: an overview of the key role of the non-bone effects. J Neuroeng Rehabil 2010;7:50.

61. Oh JH, Kim SH, Kim JH, et al. The level of vitamin D in the serum correlates with fatty degeneration of the muscles of the rotator cuff. J Bone Joint Surg Br 2009;91:1587–93.

62. Schaer M, Schober M, Berger S, et al. Biologically based strategies to augment rotator cuff tears. Int J Shoulder Surg 2012;6:51–60.

63. Angeline ME, Ma R, Pascual-Garrido C, et al. Effect of diet-induced vitamin D deficiency on rotator cuff healing in a rat model. Am J Sports Med 2014;42: 27–34.

64. Ryu KJ, Kim BH, Lee Y, et al. Low serum Vitamin D is not correlated with the severity of a rotator cuff tear or retear after arthroscopic repair. Am J Sports Med 2015;43:1743–50.

65. Tingart MJ, Apreleva M, von Stechow D, et al. The cortical thickness of the proximal humeral diaphysis predicts bone mineral density of the proximal humerus. J Bone Joint Surg Br 2003;85:611–7.

66. Boileau P, Brassart N, Watkinson DJ, et al. Arthroscopic repair of full-thickness tears of the supraspinatus: does the tendon really heal? J Bone Joint Surg Am 2005;87:1229–40.

67. Duquin TR, Buyea C, Bisson LJ. Which method of rotator cuff repair leads to the highest rate of structural healing? A systematic review. Am J Sports Med 2010;38:835–41.

68. Djurasovic M, Marra G, Arroyo JS, et al. Revision rotator cuff repair: factors influencing results. J Bone Joint Surg Am 2001;83-A:1849–55.

69. Carr A, Cooper C, Campbell MK, et al. Effectiveness of open and arthroscopic rotator cuff repair (UKUFF): a randomised controlled trial. Bone Joint J 2017;99-B:107–15.

70. Lindley K, Jones GL. Outcomes of arthroscopic versus open rotator cuff repair: a systematic review of the literature. Am J Orthop (Belle Mead NJ) 2010;39:592–600.

71. Denard PJ, Burkhart SS. Techniques for managing poor quality tissue and bone during arthroscopic rotator cuff repair. Arthroscopy 2011;27:1409–21.

72. Tauro JC. Arthroscopic "interval slide" in the repair of large rotator cuff tears. Arthroscopy 1999;15:527–30.

73. Lo IK, Burkhart SS. Arthroscopic repair of massive, contracted, immobile rotator cuff tears using single and double interval slides: technique and preliminary results. Arthroscopy 2004;20:22–33.

74. Chahal J, Mall N, MacDonald PB, et al. The role of subacromial decompression in patients undergoing arthroscopic repair of full-thickness tears of the rotator cuff: a systematic review and meta-analysis. Arthroscopy 2012;28:720–7.

75. Nathani A, Smith K, Wang T. Partial and full-thickness RCT: modern repair techniques. Curr Rev Musculoskelet Med 2018;11:113–21.

76. Kawakami J, Yamamoto N, Nagamoto H, et al. Minimum distance of suture anchors used for rotator cuff repair without decreasing the pullout strength: a biomechanical study. Arthroscopy 2018;34:377–85.

77. Lo IK, Burkhart SS. Double-row arthroscopic rotator cuff repair: re-establishing the footprint of the rotator cuff. Arthroscopy 2003;19:1035–42.

78. Park MC, Elattrache NS, Ahmad CS, et al. "Transosseous-equivalent" rotator cuff repair technique. Arthroscopy 2006;22:1360.e1-5.

79. Wang E, Wang L, Gao P, et al. Single-versus double-row arthroscopic rotator cuff repair in massive tears. Med Sci Monit 2015;21:1556–61.

80. Chen M, Xu W, Dong Q, et al. Outcomes of single-row versus double-row arthroscopic rotator cuff repair: a systematic review and meta-analysis of current evidence. Arthroscopy 2013;29:1437–49.

81. Mihata T, Watanabe C, Fukunishi K, et al. Functional and structural outcomes of single-row versus double-row versus combined double-row and suture-bridge repair for rotator cuff tears. Am J Sports Med 2011;39:2091–8.

82. Tingart MJ, Apreleva M, Lehtinen J, et al. Anchor design and bone mineral density affect the pull-out strength of suture anchors in rotator cuff repair: which anchors are best to use in patients with low bone quality? Am J Sports Med 2004;32:1466–73.

83. Milano G, Grasso A, Salvatore M, et al. Arthroscopic rotator cuff repair with metal and biodegradable suture anchors: a prospective randomized study. Arthroscopy 2010;26:S112–9.

84. Burkhart SS. The deadman theory of suture anchors: observations along a south Texas fence line. Arthroscopy 1995;11:119–23.

85. Strauss E, Frank D, Kubiak E, et al. The effect of the angle of suture anchor insertion on fixation failure at the tendon-suture interface after rotator cuff repair: deadman's angle revisited. Arthroscopy 2009;25:597–602.

86. Itoi E, Nagamoto H, Sano H, et al. Deadman theory revisited12. Biomed Mater Eng 2016;27:171–81.

87. Black EM, Austin LS, Narzikul A, et al. Comparison of implant cost and surgical time in arthroscopic transosseous and transosseous equivalent rotator cuff repair. J Shoulder Elbow Surg 2016;25:1449–56.

88. Giori NJ, Sohn DH, Mirza FM, et al. Bone cement improves suture anchor fixation. Clin Orthop Relat Res 2006;451:236–41.

89. Aziz KT, Shi BY, Okafor LC, et al. Pullout strength of standard vs. cement-augmented rotator cuff repair anchors in cadaveric bone. Clin Biomech (Bristol, Avon) 2018;54:132–6.

Foot and Ankle

Surgical Considerations for Osteoporosis in Ankle Fracture Fixation

Raymond Y. Hsu, MD[a],*, Jose M. Ramirez, MD, MA[b],
Brad D. Blankenhorn, MD[a]

KEYWORDS

- Ankle fracture • Fixation • Osteoporosis • Lateral malleolus • Medial malleolus

KEY POINTS

- The incidence of geriatric ankle fractures continues to rise.
- Fracture surgeons should be facile with multiple techniques for fixation of osteoporotic ankle fractures.
- Interfragmentary screw fixation and posterolateral antiglide plate application remains an effective fixation technique in osteoporotic fractures.
- Several techniques exist to augment traditional fixation constructs.

INTRODUCTION

As the geriatric population and orthopedic injuries in that population continues to increase,[1,2] fracture surgeons should be prepared to surgically manage osteoporotic ankle fractures. Ankle fractures in the elderly are generally not considered pathologic fragility fractures in the manner of proximal femur and distal radius fractures. Regardless of the cause of the injury, however, there are abundant challenges in the management of osteoporotic ankle fractures especially in elderly patients who have difficulty limiting weight bearing. Most osteoporosis research in foot and ankle surgery pertains to ankle fractures; however, the same lessons are applied to other foot and ankle procedures with fixation of poor-quality bone.

Primary osteoporosis is an age-related condition defined by reduced bone mineralization and increased fracture risk. Osteoporosis is characterized by loss of cancellous bone volume and

changes in the microarchitecture of bone. These changes in bone morphology alter the bone's mechanical properties.

Bone mineral density is measured based on dual-energy x-ray absorptiometry scan performed on select anatomic areas, such as the lumbar spine and the hip. The T-score, expressed in units of standard deviation, is a comparison against the average peak bone mass of a healthy young adult. Some systems compare specifically against an age of 30 years old and specify the same sex and race, whereas others do not, which can lead to confusion. According to the World Health Organization, normal bone mineral density is defined by a T score greater than or equal to −1.0. Osteopenia is defined by a T score of −1.0 to −2.5, whereas osteoporosis is defined as a T score less than or equal to −2.5.

Secondary osteoporosis is not purely age-related and is caused by underlying medical conditions.[3] These include systemic inflammatory

Disclosure statement: The authors do not have any conflicts of interest, financial or otherwise, relevant to the material presented in this article.

[a] Department of Orthopedic Surgery, The Warren Alpert Medical School at Brown University, 1 Kettle Point Avenue, East Providence, RI 02915, USA; [b] Department of Orthopedic Surgery, The Warren Alpert Medical School at Brown University, 593 Eddy Street, Providence, RI 02903, USA
* Corresponding author.
E-mail address: Raymond_Hsu@Brown.edu

conditions (ie, rheumatoid arthritis, systemic lupus erythematous); hypogonadism; endocrinopathy; diabetes mellitus; malabsorption (celiac disease, gastrectomy, pernicious anemia); chronic kidney and liver disease; and hematologic conditions, such as multiple myeloma and myeloproliferative disorders.[3] It is worthwhile for treating surgeons to be familiar with these conditions that are associated with poor bone quality. A heightened suspicion for poor bone quality may help with planning before surgery. Also, many of these underlying conditions can be treated and the osteoporosis may be at least partly reversible.

Secondary osteoporosis may also be drug induced. In this condition, a pharmacologic agent impairs bone homeostasis, ultimately leading to decreased bone mineralization[4] These medication types include glucocorticoids, selective estrogen receptor modulators, aromatase inhibitors, proton pump inhibitors, gonadotropin-releasing hormone agonists, anticonvulsants, selective serotonin reuptake inhibitors, calcineurin inhibitors, and thiazolidineiones.

CLINICAL EVIDENCE FOR FIXATION VERSUS NONOPERATIVE MANAGEMENT IN GERIATRIC PATIENTS

The objective of operative fixation of unstable ankle fractures should be to restore the anatomic and stable relationship of the tibiotalar and distal tibiofibular articulations, thereby limiting posttraumatic pain and arthritis. Ankle fractures occurring in the geriatric patient can present a technical challenge because of the osteoporotic nature of the bone and medical comorbidities. Literature suggests that geriatric ankle fractures (>age 65 years) can be performed with reliable results similar to that of younger patients.[5] Even though a high rate of return (85%) to preinjury level has been reported the general complication rate is not insignificant, ranging from 4.6% to 21%.[6–8]

Koval and colleagues[9] in a Medicare study of geriatric ankle fractures found the 1-year mortality for patients treated operatively to be 6.7% and treated nonoperatively to be 9.2%. In another Medicare study but of inpatients only, Bariteau and colleagues[10] found the 1-year mortality for geriatric patients with ankle fractures treated operatively to be 9.1% and treated nonoperatively to be 21.5%. An attempt to account for selection bias in the operative versus nonoperative groups by accounting for age and comorbidities was unable to fully account for the mortality difference in the two groups. This finding provided some indirect evidence that operative fixation may mortality benefit. Hsu and colleagues[11] showed that when compared with other geriatric patients admitted to the hospital and even after accounting for comorbidities and age differences, geriatric patients with ankle fracture admitted to the hospital demonstrated a lower 1-year mortality. This comparison suggests a greater degree of physical health in geriatric patients with ankle fracture not reflected by their age and medical history. Our general recommendation is to proceed with surgical intervention in most geriatric unstable ankle fractures. Reasons to consider nonoperative management include minimal ambulatory status, active infection or sepsis, advanced or decompensated cardiopulmonary disease, terminal illness, uncontrolled diabetes mellitus, and/or compromised soft tissue about the ankle.

Wound complications have been reported in 9% to 14% of patients[6,7] making the soft tissue envelope an important factor to consider when planning operative fixation of an osteoporotic ankle fracture. Geriatric patients can have skin that has decreased amounts of subcutaneous fat and decreased elasticity, thus making the skin less resilient and prone to injury. Diabetes mellitus and peripheral vascular disease[8,9,12] can be coincident with osteoporosis in geriatric patients, and also increase the risk of potential complications.

FIBULAR FRACTURE FIXATION

When treating distal fibular fractures, as with most periarticular fractures, the general goal is anatomic reduction, fracture compression, and adequate stabilization. As an exception, bridging constructs are used or comminuted fractures when anatomic reduction and fixation would cause too much additional injury or is impossible. For the typical oblique fracture, our preference is to place the fibular plate in the posterolateral antiglide position with interfragmentary screws placed through the plate if possible.[13] Although the antiglide plate construct can be used to reduce the distal fracture fragment into the proper position, with osteoporotic bone there is a risk of further comminution with this technique. Our preference in osteoporotic bone is to first achieve reduction and provisional fixation before plate application. Using a bone spreader to achieve distraction and length in an osteoporotic fibula fracture may at times be too destructive. We find a Hintermann or K-wire distractor with the wires placed well proximal and distal to the fracture site to be particularly useful in these situations to slowly distract the fracture before reduction without comminuting the fracture line. As shown by Shymon and Harris,[14] K-wires and a toothed lamina spreader are used as a low-cost alternative to the Hintermann distractor. We typically perform initial fracture reduction with the aid of pointed reduction clamps. Interfragmentary screws of 2.7 or 3.5 mm are inserted in lag or positional technique before plate application if the bone is amenable. **Fig. 1** demonstrates fibular fixation in a 70-year-old patient with osteoporosis (see **Fig. 1A, B**). Given the patient's poor bone quality, the distal fibula was fixed with a positional interfragmentary screw followed by application of an antiglide plate (see **Fig. 1C, D**). In poor-quality bone, where compression is already sufficiently achieved by reduction clamps, a positional as opposed to a lag screw has the advantage of having threads on both sides of the fracture line. In osteoporotic bone, relying only on the interface between the screw head and thin cortex for even preliminary fixation on the over-drilled side of the fracture is prone to loss of fixation and iatrogenic comminution.

The advantages of the posterior antiglide plate over direct lateral plating include less bending of the plate and placement of much longer distal screws without screw penetration of the joint. More importantly, biomechanically, lateral plating has been shown to be an inferior construct when directly compared with posterior antiglide plating in osteoporotic bone.[15,16]

Posterior plating can also be advantageous in elderly individuals because it prevents the hardware from lying subcutaneously as it would with lateral plating[17] perhaps reducing the chances of wound complications. Posterior plating, however, has been associated with peroneal tendon irritation and symptomatic hardware removal in up to 18% of patients.[18] Another series by Weber and Krause[19] found similar results but the authors also completed a cadaveric study and concluded that peroneal irritation could be mostly avoided by limiting how distal the plate extends and not filling the most distal screw hole if the plate does extend.

LOCKED PLATING

Locking technology for fixation of osteoporotic distal fibular fractures has gained additional credence over the last decade. Zahn and colleagues[20] demonstrated in a cadaveric biomechanical model that locked lateral plating is superior to nonlocked lateral plating for the fixation of osteoporotic fibular fractures. However, Minihane and colleagues[15] in another cadaveric study demonstrated that posterior antiglide plating with a one-third tubular plate is biomechanically superior to lateral fixation with a locked one-third tubular plate. Importantly, the locking construct used in this investigation included just two screws in the distal fracture segment. Newer locking distal fibula plates have multiple (>2) distal screw options.

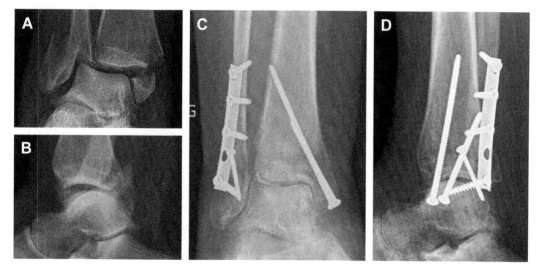

Fig. 1. (*A, B*) A 70-year-old woman's injury and (*C, D*) 11-week follow-up standing radiographs of her unstable tri-malleolar ankle fracture. Fixation started medially and poor bone quality was confirmed and addressed with bicortical positional screws. Lateral fixation was accomplished with a positional (instead of lagged) interfragmentary screw and an antiglide plate.

Fig. 2 demonstrates the injury radiographs and postoperative radiographs in a 71-year-old woman with osteoporosis. A variable angle locking plate was used in fixation of the distal fibular fracture.

The 2016 meta-analysis by Dingemans and colleagues[21] evaluated the biomechanical properties of different distal fibular plating options. Their meta-analysis permitted a comparison of lateral unlocked and locked plating only. They did not find any significant differences between the two constructs with regard to torsional stiffness or torque to failure. The authors conclude that lateral locked plating may not be biomechanically superior to lateral conventional plating, which they believe may be caused by decreased frictional forces and rigidity seen with precontoured locked plating because the bone is not compressed to the plate. However, the biomechanical properties of locked plating were found to be independent of bone mineral density representing a theoretic advantage in patients with osteoporosis. Authors highlight that several less expensive options for fibular fixation exist including posterolateral antiglide plating, which may be a suitable alterative for fixation in the elderly. Lastly, studies have demonstrated a higher rate of wound complications associated with locking plates when compared with nonlocking plates.[22]

A more recent cadaveric investigation, published after the previously mentioned meta-analysis, directly compared posterior antiglide plating and newer locked periarticular plating constructs (with multiple screw options in the distal fragment) in the fixation of osteoporotic fibular fractures.[23] The authors reported a significantly higher torque-to-failure and construct stiffness with locked plating. Locked plates failed via fragmentation of the distal fibula through the cluster of screws in the distal aspect of the plate. The authors theorize that multiple screws in the distal segment may weaken the already osteoporotic bone. However, they did note that the torque-to-failure in the locked plating specimens exceeded the torque to failure in the antiglide specimens.

Hereafter we present several other viable surgical techniques and considerations to be made when managing osteoporotic ankle fractures.

INTRAMEDULLARY K-WIRE AUGMENTATION

One of the salient properties of osteoporotic bone is a loss of trabecular volume. Screws traversing these bones achieve less purchase with the bone and exhibit less torsional stiffness and pullout strength when compared with placement in nonosteoporotic bone.

In the intramedullary wire technique two smooth 1.2-mm K-wires are inserted in a retrograde fashion into the medullary canal of the fibula after reduction is achieved. The wires are advanced to a level just proximal to the end of the plate that is going to be used. Fig. 3 demonstrates uses of this technique in a 67-year-old woman with an osteoporotic ankle fracture. Insertion of cortical screws proceeds in standard fashion. Each hole is drilled through the lateral

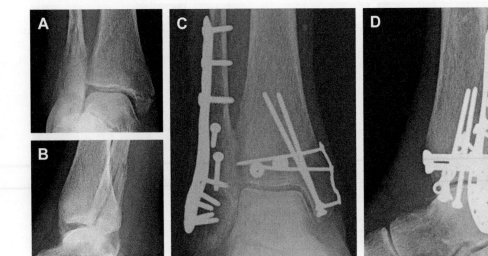

Fig. 2. (A, B) Injury and (C, D) 4-month follow-up standing radiographs of a comminuted ankle fracture in a 71-year-old woman with osteoporosis that failed initial nonoperative management. The fibular fixation was reinforced with a variable angle locking plate.

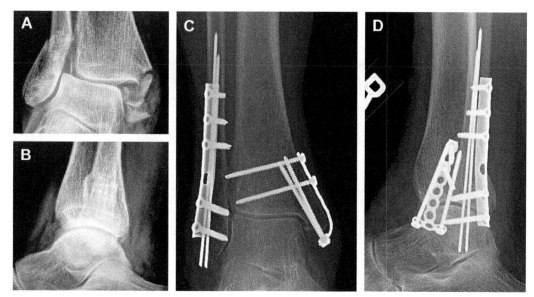

Fig. 3. (A, B) Injury and (C, D) 9-month follow-up standing radiographs of a 67-year-old woman's comminuted ankle fracture. The fibular fixation was reinforced with 1.2-mm intramedullary K-wires with interdigitating screws from a posterior lateral plate. The medial comminution was addressed with a contoured 2.4-mm T-plate with 2.7-mm screws.

cortex and through the pin "traffic" in the canal and finally through the medial cortex. Care should be taken to clamp the wires before drilling and screw placement because the wires otherwise can be wrapped up and driven more proximally than desired. Koval and colleagues[24] have reported good outcomes (89% with either no, slight, or moderate pain) in a 20-patient series that underwent fixation of osteoporotic fractures with this technique. As corollary they performed a biomechanical comparison of this technique with conventional fibular plating with a one-third tubular plate. Bending and torsional resistance was found to be significantly greater with K-wire augmentation.

Assal and colleagues[25] have reported their outcomes using a combined intramedullary wire with cement augmentation technique. They report a preferred technique wherein a 2.5-mm threaded wire is passed retrograde from the tip for the lateral malleolus to the junction of the middle and distal one-third of the fibula. A lateral neutralization plate is then placed with polymethyl methacrylate (PMMA) injected into the screw holes before insertion. Thirty-six patients with a mean age of 79.2 were included in the study. All fractures healed without loss of reduction and they reported that 90% of patients were able to return to prefracture function.

Dunn and colleagues[26] reported the biomechanical results of another additional modification

of this technique for osteoporotic fibular fractures. In their technique, the intramedullary canal is again augmented with smooth K-wires. Additionally, the proximal screws in the plate are inserted in tetra-cortical fashion through both cortices in the fibula and tibia. When compared with a lateral plate with intramedullary K-wires, the technique with quadricortical screws was stiffer and more resistant to axial load.

DOUBLE/STACKED PLATING

Dual plate fixation is a low-cost technique for adding stability by increasing stiffness in complex or osteoporotic fibular fractures. In the stacked plating technique, two one-third tubular plates are stacked together and then fixed onto bone (**Fig. 4**). In normal-quality bone without comminution, there is sufficient intrinsic stability at the bone-bone interface with compression that a flexible neutralization plate is adequate and the stiffness of the system is determined by the bone. In comminuted fractures or osteoporotic fractures, the intrinsic stability of the fracture is lacking and the stiffness of the system is dictated by the stiffness of the plating system. From a failure perspective, with a flexible plate on osteoporotic bone, there is enough flexibility in the system that a bone-screw interface can fail before the adjacent one fails. With a more rigid plate, although not as stiff as a fixed angle device, complete failure at a bone-screw interface

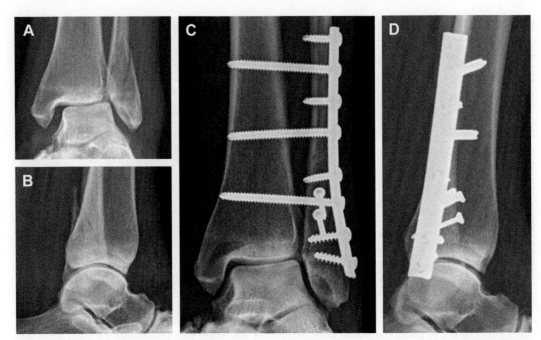

Fig. 4. (A, B) Injury standing and (C, D) 12-week follow-up standing radiographs of an unstable distal fibula fracture in a 67-year-old woman with insulin-dependent diabetes, neuropathy, and chronic steroid use for pulmonary disease. A stiffer construct was accomplished with two stacked one-third-tubular plates and multiple syndesmotic screws.

cannot occur without some compromise at an adjacent interface.

Alternatively, two plates in a near 90-to-90 orientation are used to achieve rigid stabilization of the fracture. Fig. 5 demonstrates the injury radiographs of a 74-year-old man with diabetic nephropathy who sustained a displaced ankle fracture after a ground level fall. A posterolateral one-third tubular antiglide plate with additional fixation into the tibia with 3.5-mm cortical screws was used. Despite this, there was noted motion at the fracture site, so a second quarter tubular plate was placed anterolaterally on the fibula. After four additional screws were inserted in an anteroposterior direction, no motion was noted at the fracture site while the ankle joint was passively taken through range of motion. This technique is again demonstrated in Fig. 6 with a secondary six-hole locking one-third tubular plate.

Vance and Vosseller[27] retrospectively reviewed 12 cases of patients with distal fibular fractures treated with dual, biplanar plating. The average patient age was 51 years of age (range, 20–83) and four of the patients carried a diagnosis of osteoporosis and two were diabetic with neuropathy. At a mean time of 25.6 months postoperative, all 12 fractures had healed. Ten of 12 patients denied any hardware-related symptoms

and reported good Foot and Ankle Outcome Score with regard to activities of daily living (90.4; standard deviation, 14.5) and sports (89.5; standard deviation, 18.1).

CEMENT AUGMENTATION

Use of cement is another technique for increasing the density of the intramedullary canal thereby increasing the purchase of inserted screws. In this technique, the cement is mixed and injected into the medullary canal of the distal fibula and allowed to harden while the fracture is held reduced with reduction clamps. After the cement has hardened, the fibula and cement are drilled and screws inserted in standard fashion.

Cement augmentation does offer some advantage over cancellous autografting. This includes decreased risk of donor site morbidity and offering a higher degree of stability to the construct at the time of fixation.[28] PMMA, widely used in orthopedics, is one compound that is used for augmentation. Potential drawbacks to using PMMA for fracture fixation include its inability to be resorbed, the amount of heat generated as it cures, and the difficulty of removal in the setting of revision or infection.[28] Several calcium phosphate cements are

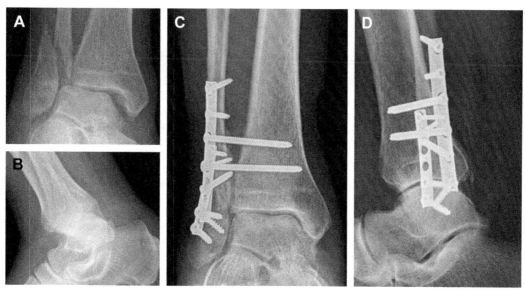

Fig. 5. (*A*, *B*) Injury and (*C*, *D*) 13-week follow-up standing radiographs of an unstable ankle fracture in a 74-year-old man with diabetic neuropathy. Comminution and bone quality prevented stable fibular fixation with an antiglide plate alone. Fixation was reinforced with a lateral quarter-tubular plate and quadricortical syndesmotic screws.

commercially available. Calcium phosphate cures with compressive strengths similar to bone yet it has been shown to have osteoinductive properties, and, unlike PMMA, it is resorbed over time.[29]

Panchbhavi and colleagues[30] evaluated the biomechanical properties of cement augmentation on screw performance. In their cadaveric study they inserted 4.0-mm cancellous screws into a distal fibula after augmenting the holes with an injected mixture of calcium phosphate and calcium sulfate. They observed a 240% increased force needed to pull out and a 450% increase in energy absorbed before pull out compared with nonaugmented screws. However, the stiffness to pullout did not change with

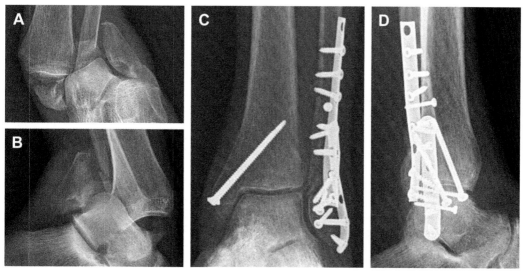

Fig. 6. (*A*, *B*) Injury and (*C*, *D*) 14-week follow-up standing radiographs of an ankle fracture dislocation in a 66-year-old man with hypovitaminosis D and chronic steroid use for pulmonary disease. Fixation started with bicortical positional screws for the less comminuted medial malleolus. The lateral malleolus was addressed with positional interfragmentary screws and a posterior lateral plate. The construct was not stable until the addition of a locking one-third-tubular plate.

cement augmentation. They intuit that added holding power afforded by the cement and bone interface may be dependent on bone quality because energy to pullout trended upward with increased bone density.

Panchbhavi and colleagues[31] performed a follow-up biomechanical study wherein they examined external rotation, torque, stiffness, and energy absorbed at failure in paired osteoporotic cadavers with a simulated fibular osteotomy fixed with a locked plate. They were unable to replicate the significant differences when comparing augmented and nonaugmented constructs. They theorize that the locked configuration creates a fixed angle device with different mechanical properties not impacted by cementing and hypothesize that nonlocking screws may have produced larger observed differences.

TIBIA PRO FIBULA

Insertion of syndesmotic or so-called tibia-pro-fibula screws is another way to augment fixation of osteoporotic fractures. Fixation into the tibia provides cortical and trabecular purchase to the constructs. Biomechanical data performed in the context of syndesmotic disruption does not identify any differences in fibular displacement or force on the fibula with ankle dorsiflexion or external rotation with the use of screws 3.5 versus 4.5 mm diameter or tricortical versus quadricortical purchase.[32] When used to augment fixation of an osteoporotic fibular fracture, as shown in **Fig. 4**, our practice is to insert 3.5-mm cortical screws in a quadricortical fashion into the medial and lateral cortices of the tibia as a means to increase screw purchase in a nonlocked plate construct. A recent biomechanical cadaveric study of osteoporotic distal fibular fixation evaluated the effect of augmenting a locked plating construct with tibia-pro-fibula screws. Augmentation in the locked plate setting did not produce significant mechanical differences.[31]

Especially in the setting of osteoporotic bone, care needs to be taken to not overtighten these syndesmotic screws. In good-quality bone, the screw stops when the screw head hits the plate. With overtightening in poor-quality bone or a comminuted fibula, the screw threads obtain better purchase in the tibia and strip the bone in the fibula. The screw head then continues to advance despite hitting the plate and pulls the plate as a washer and displaces the fibula fracture.

INTRAMEDULLARY NAILING

Intramedullary nailing of distal fibula fractures is another option for the management of distal fibula fractures. Nail insertion and reduction is performed under fluoroscopy and thus requires considerably less soft tissue dissection[33] when compared with open reduction and internal fixation. Intramedullary fixation may be an attractive option if the soft tissue about the posterolateral distal fibula is compromised or threatened because this avoids a surgical incision and/or plate prominence in this area. Some authors note that transverse, length stable fractures may be best suited for intramedullary nailing, whereas open, comminuted and very distal fractures of the fibula are not indicated for intramedullary fixation.[34] Additionally, syndesmotic fixation in unstable ankle fractures is accomplished through the implant.[34]

Biomechanical data support the use of intramedullary fibular nailing in unstable ankle fracture patterns.[23,35] In one recent study Smith and colleagues[35] performed a study on osteoporotic cadavers (average age of 82 years) wherein SER IV, bimalleolar injury patterns were simulated and fixed with either an interfragmentary screw and plate construct or an intramedullary nail. They found a higher torque to failure in the intramedullary nail group. Importantly, while screw and plate construct all failed via screw pullout, the intramedullary nail construct failed via lateral ligament disruption.

Early clinical data on the intramedullary nailing in osteoporotic ankle fracture is reassuring.[36] Ramasamy and Sherry[36] reported good and excellent results in 11 patients (average age, 67.2) treated with Weber type B ankle fractures. In 2018, Jordan and colleagues[37] performed a systematic review of intramedullary nailing of the fibula. They identified 10 studied evaluating the outcomes of fibular fixation with an intramedullary device. The preponderance of studies were low-level case reports and only two studies were clinical case series. In a prospective randomized trial Asloum and colleagues[38] compared plate fixation with intramedullary nailing in 71 patients (mean age, 53 ± 19). They reported no statistically significant differences in bony union; yet the intramedullary group had a significantly lower (7% vs 56%) rate of complication and significantly better functional outcomes. Skin necrosis was the most common complication of the plate fixation group. Although high-level comparative studies are lacking, intramedullary nailing of fibular fractures has produced acceptable outcomes with low rates of complication and may be indicated in the elderly comorbid patient.[37]

We do not routinely use intramedullary fibular nails in our practice. In certain instances, soft tissue envelope about the lateral malleolus may preclude open reduction and internal fixation. In that situation, we have, anecdotally, been able to successfully manage distal fibular fractures with minimal displacement with the insertion of long 3.5-mm screws in the medullary canal of the fibula. This is performed in retrograde fashion via a stab incision over the distal tip of the fibula. This technique is seen in **Fig. 7**, which demonstrates injury radiographs and postoperative radiographs of a 70-year-old woman who sustained a left ankle fracture. A soft tissue injury over the lateral malleolus prevented open reduction and plating, thus the fibular fracture alignment was held percutaneously and a retrograde 3.5-mm cortical screw was inserted.

We believe that the single intramedullary screw technique is best used when the risks of an open reduction and plate outweigh the benefits of an anatomic reduction but some additional lateral stability is desired. Especially after stability has already been mostly restored with medial fixation, a lateral intramedullary screw may not restore lateral anatomy but allows the fibula to provide some additional resistance to lateral talar translation. With screw insertion, as the proximal screw engages the medial cortex of the fibula and the thinner diaphysis, the distal screw medializes the distal fibular fragment, providing additional stability.

MEDIAL MALLEOLAR FIXATION
Transverse or Oblique Fractures
Unicortical fixation with partially threaded 4.0-mm cancellous screws is a long established technique fixation for transverse and oblique medial malleolar fractures.[39] Although compression of the fracture is achieved inherently by this lag-by-design technique, as with all interfragmentary screw techniques, the stiffness and resistance to failure of the construct is reliant on the purchase on both sides of the fracture. Purchase of the distal fragment with lag screw fixation relies substantially on the screw head interface with the cortex because there are no threads purchasing the distal fracture fragment. Additionally, proximal, metaphyseal fixation is reliant on the quality of the distal cancellous bone of the tibia. With osteoporotic bone, especially with comminution, unicortical lag screws may not be the best technique for obtaining a stable fixation construct. Because transverse and oblique medial malleolar fractures generally fail in tension, the fixation construct is reliant on the pull-out strength of the proximal screw threads in osteoporotic cancellous bone and of the distal osteoporotic fragment around the screw heads.

The traditional alternative for fixation of transverse medial malleolar fractures is a tension band wire construct.[39] Tension band wiring has been specifically advocated for osteoporotic bone.[40,41] For compression of the fracture site, a tension band wire construct relies on reasonable bone quality and intact bone at the fracture line for compression to occur. In resisting displacement, any tension deforming forces on

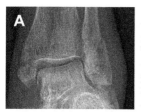
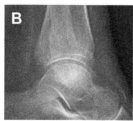
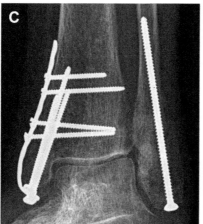
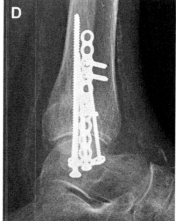

Fig. 7. A 70-year-old woman's (*A*, *B*) injury and (*C*, *D*) 6-week follow-up standing radiographs of her left ankle fracture. Comminution of the medial malleolus was addressed with a contoured 2.4-mm T-plate with 2.7-mm screws distally. Because of soft tissue damage laterally, fibular stability was accomplished with percutaneous manipulation and an intramedullary 3.5-mm screw in lieu of open plating.

the distal fragment are transmitted proximally through the tension wire instead of directly through the interfragmentary fixation. In a prospective consecutive series of 31 fractures by Ostrum and Litsky,[40] there were no nonunions and in a biomechanical study in the same paper, tension band wiring was demonstrated to be superior to cancellous screws with respect to resisting pronation forces. Tension band wiring is a good option for osteoporotic medial malleolar fractures but still requires reasonable bone quality and minimal comminution to allow sufficient capture and provisional maintenance of reduction by the distal wires. There is also a notable issue of subcutaneous hardware prominence.[40,41] Thin skin overlying the medial concave flare and supramalleolar portions of the distal tibia in geriatric patients may preclude the use of a tension band.

Bicortical interfragmentary screw fixation (see Figs. 1, 2, and 7; Fig. 8) for transverse or oblique medial malleolar fractures as opposed to unicortical fixation is particularly useful for osteoporotic fractures.[42,43] The use of cortical fully threaded screws that engage the far cortex offers better proximal purchase with greater thread count, longer screws, and capture of denser cortical bone, all without the subcutaneous hardware of a tension band or plate. Ricci and colleagues[44] performed a retrospective comparison of 46 fractures fixed with two unicortical 4.0-mm cancellous lag screws and 46

fractures fixed with two bicortical 3.5-mm cortical lag screws. The unicortical fixation group demonstrated higher rates of radiographic loosening (24% vs 2%) and a higher rate of nonunion (2 vs 0) yet were minimally symptomatic. Their cadaveric biomechanical study of screw purchase as determined by maximal torque before stripping the bone confirmed greater purchase with bicortical screws.[44] Fowler and colleagues[45] similarly demonstrated in a sawbones mechanical study that bicortical screws created a stiffer fixation construct than unicortical screws or a tension band.

We advocate for the use of bicortical fixation of medial malleolar fractures whenever bone quality is a concern with two 3.5-mm or 2.7-mm screws depending on the size of the fracture fragment. Both screws are started at the anterior colliculus to avoid irritation of the posterior tibial tendon that can occur with more posterior starting points. When possible, the screws are diverged for greater spread at the fracture site and improved rotational stability. This is especially true for 2.7-mm screws, which are not generally available in longer screw lengths. The screw trajectories are directed somewhat posteriorly to obtain bicortical purchase without necessitating an exceedingly long screw. Furthermore, after adequate compression is obtained with reduction clamps, screws are placed in positional configuration without overdrilling the distal fragment. This preserves thread

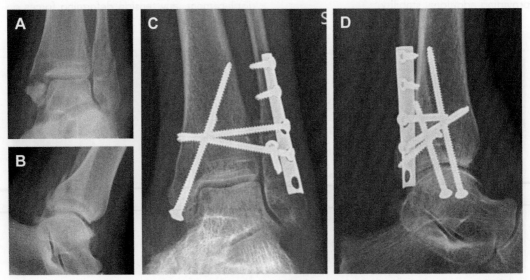

Fig. 8. A 66-year-old woman's (A, B) injury and (C, D) 15-week follow-up standing radiographs of her unstable trimalleolar ankle fracture. Bone quality assessed during placement of the fibular lag screw and antiglide plate prompted use of bicortical medial malleolar positional screws and quadricortical syndesmotic screws for additional fixation.

purchase of the distal fragment. Parker and colleagues[46] used pressure sensing film to examine fracture compression in a medial malleolus cadaver study. They found that fully threaded screws placed with only the initial compression from reduction clamps maintained greater compression of the fracture site than similarly placed lag screws by either technique or design.

Vertical Fractures

Vertically oriented medial malleolar fractures fail in axial load or shear instead of tension and are generally fixed with lag screws perpendicular to the fracture, an antiglide plate, or an antiglide plate with additional lag screws through the plate.[39,47,48] Toolan and colleagues[48] demonstrated in a biomechanical study that for vertical medial malleolar fractures, two transverse 4.0-mm cancellous lag screws placed perpendicularly across the fracture are superior to the same lag screws placed obliquely up the medial malleolus. They also found that two independent transverse lag screws were superior to a one-third tubular antiglide plate with either only two 3.5-mm proximal screws or with a single additional lag 3.5-mm screw right below the apex crossing the fracture.[48] An antiglide plate extending more distally with multiple lag or positional screws through the plate and across the fracture was not examined. In subsequent biomechanical studies, Dumigan and colleagues[49] and Wegner and colleagues[47] examined a one-third tubular antiglide plate that extends more distally and includes two 3.5-mm transverse distal screws through the plate. Both studies found that this more robust antiglide construct was mechanically superior when compared with independent transverse screw constructs of either two 4.0-mm cancellous lag screws or two 3.5-mm cortical bicortical screws.[47,49] Fig. 9 shows the use of a long medial plate construct with multiple screws in the distal fracture fragment.

With osteoporotic bone, when the soft tissue envelope permits, use of an antiglide plate that extends distally and includes multiple distal transverse bicortical screws through the plate is advisable to better counter deforming forces across a broader bone and metal interface. The benefit of additional compression with lag by technique of the distal screws has to be weighed against the benefit of better purchase of the distal fragment with positional unlagged screws. Also, with osteoporotic bone, more precontouring of the plate should be completed before placement because an undercontoured plate may displace the fracture or comminute the distal fragment.

Comminuted Fractures

Comminuted osteoporotic medial malleolar fractures are especially challenging. Medial malleolar fractures that are essentially a traditionally described horizontal, oblique, or vertical fracture but with marginal comminution at the cortex and articular surface may complicate reduction. These can generally still be fixed, however, with bicortical screws or an antiglide plate, respectively. There are a subset of comminuted fractures that have substantial additional coronal and sagittal plane fracture lines or even be a variant that involves extension into posterior medial plafond.[50] In average bone quality, these can sometimes be pieced together with interfragmentary fixation, but with osteoporotic bone, independent screws may have insufficient purchase. Especially in the setting of osteoporotic bone and fracture dislocations, these comminuted fractures can be grossly unstable in tension and axial load. Fixation in this setting may benefit from a construct that even if unable to anatomically compress each fracture line, supports overall alignment against tension and axial load failure.

As shown in **Fig. 3**, soft tissue permitting, a 2.0-mm or 2.4-mm T-plate can be contoured to sit medially over the distal tibia and wrapped distally directly over the superficial deltoid origin over the anterior colliculus. This plate placement allows for multiple interfragmentary screws from distal to proximal across the main fracture line through the plate even through comminution and the distal plate acts as a distal buttress or washer against loss of fixation. The extension of the plate proximally resists axial and tension loads. Amanatullah and colleagues[51] found a 2.0-mm T-plate construct with 2.0-mm screws distally and proximally to be a stiffer construct than either two 4.0-mm unicortical lag screws or a wire tension band. For additional fixation, a 2.4-mm T-plate permits the use of longer 2.7-mm screws distally, which again can be aimed proximally and posteriorly to obtain a bicortical purchase. The overall construct combines aspects of bicortical fixation with tension band technique. Care should be taken to ensure that the soft tissue envelope permits placement of this construct.

MEDICAL CONSIDERATIONS

Although vitamin D is part of the medical armamentarium for the prevention and management

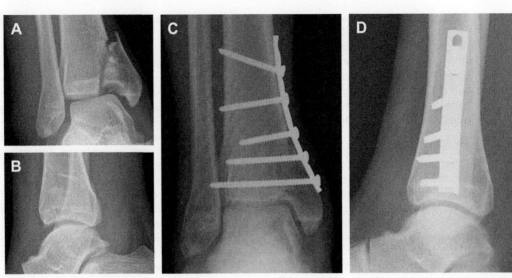

Fig. 9. (*A*, *B*) Injury and (*C*, *D*) 6-month follow-up standing radiographs of a vertical medial malleolar fracture. Biomechanical studies support the use of an antiglide plate that extends more distally and multiple distal screws through the plate that cross the fracture.

of osteoporosis, its role in fracture healing remains to be definitely elucidated.[52,53] Several clinical studies have reported a positive effect of vitamin D on extremity fracture healing.[54,55] For example, a Danish study by Doetsch and colleagues,[54] evaluated the effects of vitamin D supplementation on proximal humerus fracture healing and bone mineral density in a placebo randomized clinical trial of 30 women with osteoporosis. They demonstrated increased deposit of fracture callus at 6 weeks in the vitamin D supplementation group. More recently, Gorter and colleagues[52] concluded in a larger retrospective study of extremity fractures that vitamin D level at the time of fracture may indeed influence fracture healing. In their study they report a clinical nonunion rate of 9.7% in the vitamin deficient group compared with 0.3% in the group that was not deficient at the time of fracture. A recent study conducted in mice found only a marginal effect of vitamin D on fracture healing.[56] However, the authors did find that vitamin D supplementation begun after a fracture effectively prevented post-traumatic bone loss in the intact mouse skeleton. This suggests that post-fixation supplementation of vitamin D may allow the bone to mineralize the fracture without a net loss in total body calcium and further decreasing bone mineral density.

Our standard practice is to check vitamin D levels in the perioperative setting. Patients with serum 25-hydroxy vitamin D levels of 20 to 30 ng/mL are started on daily supplementation with a daily goal of 800 to 1000 IU from prescription and dietary sources. Vitamin D–deficient patients with serum levels less than 20 ng/mL are started on weekly replacement with 50,000 IU for 8 weeks.

SUMMARY

The incidence of osteoporotic ankle fractures will increase with an aging and active population. Traditional fixation techniques alone may not be sufficient for use in osteoporotic bone. Fracture surgeons should be facile with a variety of surgical techniques, such as the ones presented here, which can be used to optimize outcomes of these fractures.

REFERENCES

1. Kannus P, Palvanen M, Niemi S, et al. Increasing number and incidence of low-trauma ankle fractures in elderly people. Finnish statistics during 1970–2000 and projections for the future. Bone 2002;31:430–3.
2. Koval K, Lurie J, Zhou W, et al. Ankle fractures in the elderly: what you get depends on where you live and who you see. J Orthop Trauma 2005;19: 635–9.
3. Sheu A, Diamond T. Secondary osteoporosis. Aust Prescr 2016;39:85–7.
4. Panday K, Gona A, Humphrey MB. Medication-induced osteoporosis: screening and treatment strategies. Ther Adv Musculoskel Dis 2014;6: 185–202.
5. Ehrenfreund T, Haluzan D, Dobric I, et al. Operative management of unstable ankle fractures in the

elderly: our institutional experience. Injury 2013;44: S20–2.

6. Srinivasan C, Moran C. Internal fixation of ankle fractures in the very elderly. Inj Int J Care Inj 2001; 32:559–63.

7. Varenne Y, Curado J, Asloum Y, et al. Analysis of risk factors of the postoperative complications of surgical treatment of ankle fractures in the elderly: a series of 477 patients. Orthop Traumatol Surg Res 2016;102S:S245–8.

8. Zaghloul A, Haddad B, Barksfield R, et al. Early complications of surgery in operative treatment of ankle fractures in those over 60: a review of 186 cases. Injury 2014;45:780–3.

9. Koval K, Zhou W, Sparks MJ, et al. Complications after ankle fracture in elderly patients. Foot Ankle Int 2007;28:1249–55.

10. Bariteau J, Hsu RY, Mor V, et al. Operative versus nonoperative treatment of geriatric ankle fractures: a Medicare Part A claims database analysis. Foot Ankle Int 2015;36:648–55.

11. Hsu R, Lee Y, Hayda R, et al. Morbidity and mortality associated with geriatric ankle fractures: a Medicare Part A claims database analysis. J Bone Joint Surg Am 2015;97:1748–55.

12. SooHoo N, Krenek L, Eagan MJ, et al. Complication rates following open reduction and internal fixation of ankle fractures. J Bone Joint Surg Am 2009; 91:1042–9.

13. Ostrum RF. Posterior plating of displaced weber B fibula fractures. J Orthop Trauma 1996;10:199–203.

14. Shymon S, Harris T. Low-cost intra-articular distraction technique using Kirschner wires and a toothed lamina spreader. J Foot Ankle Surg 2017;56:605–8.

15. Minihane K, Lee C, Ahn C, et al. Comparison of lateral locking plate and antiglide plate for fixation of distal fibular fractures in osteoporotic bone: a biomechanical study. J Orthop Trauma 2006;20: 562–6.

16. Schaffer J, Manoli A. The antiglide plate for distal fibular fixation. A biomechanical comparison with fixation with a lateral plate. J Bone Joint Surg Am 1987;69:596–604.

17. Rammelt S. Management of ankle fractures in the elderly. EOR 2016;1:239–46.

18. Vance D, Swindell H, Greisberg J, et al. Outcomes following posterior and posterolateral plating of distal fibula fractures. Foot Ankle Spec 2018. 1938640018788433. [Epub ahead of print].

19. Weber M, Krause F. Peroneal tendon lesions caused by antiglide plates used for fixation of lateral malleolar fractures: the effect of plate and screw position. Foot Ankle Int 2005;26:281–5.

20. Zahn R, Frey S, Jakubietz R. A contoured locking plate for distal fibular fractures in osteoporotic bone: a biomechanical cadaver study. Injury 2012; 43:718–25.

21. Dingemans SA, Lodeizen OAP, Goslings JC, et al. Reinforced fixation of distal fibula fractures in elderly patients; a meta-analysis of biomechanical studies. Clin Biomech Bristol Avon 2016;36:14–20.

22. Schepers T, Lieshout E, Vries M, et al. Increased rates of wound complications with locking plates in distal fibular fractures. Injury 2011;42:1125–9.

23. Switaj PJ, Wetzel RJ, Jain NP, et al. Comparison of modern locked plating and antiglide plating for fixation of osteoporotic distal fibular fractures. Foot Ankle Surg Off J Eur Soc Foot Ankle Surg 2016; 22:158–63.

24. Koval KJ, Petraco DM, Kummer FJ, et al. A new technique for complex fibula fracture fixation in the elderly: a clinical and biomechanical evaluation. J Orthop Trauma 1997;11:28–33.

25. Assal M, Christofilopoulos P, Lübbeke A, et al. Increased rates of wound complications with locking plates in distal fibular fractures. J Orthop Trauma 2011;25:742–7.

26. Dunn WR, Easley ME, Parks BG, et al. An augmented fixation method for distal fibular fractures in elderly patients: a biomechanical evaluation. Foot Ankle Int 2004;25:128–31.

27. Vance DD, Vosseller JT. Double plating of distal fibula fractures. Foot Ankle Spec 2017;10:543–6.

28. Larsson S. Cement augmentation in fracture treatment. Scand J Surg 2006;95:111–8.

29. Elder S, Frankenburg E, Goulet J. Biomechanical evaluation of calcium phosphate cement-augmented fixation of unstable intertrochanteric fractures. J Orthop Trauma 2000;14:386–93.

30. Panchbhavi V, Vallurupalli S, Morris R, et al. The use of calcium sulfate and calcium phosphate composite graft to augment screw purchase in osteoporotic ankles. Foot Ankle Int 2008;29:593–600.

31. Panchbhavi V, Vallurupalli S, Morris R. Comparison of augmentation methods for internal fixation of osteoporotic ankle fractures. Foot Ankle Int 2009; 30:696–703.

32. Markolf K, Jackson S, McAllister D. Syndesmosis fixation using dual 3.5 mm and 4.5 mm screws with tricortical and quadricortical purchase: a biomechanical study. Foot Ankle Int 2013;34:734–9.

33. Bugler K, Watson C, Hardie A. The treatment of unstable fractures of the ankle using the Acumed fibular nail: development of a technique. J Bone Joint Surg Br 2012;94:1107–12.

34. Walton D, Adams S, Parekh S. Intramedullary fixation for fractures of the distal fibula. Foot Ankle Int 2016;37:115–23.

35. Smith G, Mackenzie S, Wallace R, et al. Biomechanical comparison of intramedullary fibular nail versus plate and screw fixation. Foot Ankle Int 2017;38: 1394–9.

36. Ramasamy P, Sherry P. The role of a fibular nail in the management of Weber type B ankle fractures

in elderly patients with osteoporotic bone: a preliminary report. Inj Int J Care Inj 2001;32:477–85.

37. Jordan R, Champman A, Buchanan D, et al. The role of intramedullary fixation in ankle fractures: a systematic review. Foot Ankle Surg 2018;24: 1–10.

38. Asloum Y, Bedin B, Roger T, et al. Internal fixation of the fibula in ankle fractures. A prospective, randomized and comparative study: plating versus nailing. Orthop Traumatol Surg Res 2014;100: S255–9.

39. Ebraheim NA, Ludwig T, Weston JT, et al. Comparison of surgical techniques of 111 medial malleolar fractures classified by fracture geometry. Foot Ankle Int 2014;35:471–7.

40. Ostrum RF, Litsky AS. Tension band fixation of medial malleolus fractures. J Orthop Trauma 1992;6:464–8.

41. Georgiadis GM, White DB. Modified tension band wiring of medial malleolar ankle fractures. Foot Ankle Int 1995;16:64–8.

42. Parada SA, Krieg JC, Benirschke SK, et al. Bicortical fixation of medial malleolar fractures. Am J Orthop Belle Mead NJ 2013;42:90–2.

43. Kupcha P, Pappas S. Medial malleolar fixation with a bicortical screw: technique tip. Foot Ankle Int 2008;29:1151–3.

44. Ricci WM, Tornetta P, Borrelli J. Lag screw fixation of medial malleolar fractures: a biomechanical, radiographic, and clinical comparison of unicortical partially threaded lag screws and bicortical fully threaded lag screws. J Orthop Trauma 2012;26: 602–6.

45. Fowler TT, Pugh KJ, Litsky AS, et al. Medial malleolar fractures: a biomechanical study of fixation techniques. Orthopedics 2011;34:e349–55.

46. Parker L, Garlick N, McCarthy I, et al. Screw fixation of medial malleolar fractures: a cadaveric biomechanical study challenging the current AO philosophy. Bone Jt J 2013;95–B:1662–6.

47. Wegner AM, Wolinsky PR, Robbins MA, et al. Antiglide plating of vertical medial malleolus fractures provides stiffer initial fixation than bicortical or unicortical screw fixation. Clin Biomech Bristol Avon 2016;31:29–32.

48. Toolan BC, Koval KJ, Kummer FJ, et al. Vertical shear fractures of the medial malleolus: a biomechanical study of five internal fixation techniques. Foot Ankle Int 1994;15:483–9.

49. Dumigan RM, Bronson DG, Early JS. Analysis of fixation methods for vertical shear fractures of the medial malleolus. J Orthop Trauma 2006;20: 687–91.

50. Weber M. Trimalleolar fractures with impaction of the posteromedial tibial plafond: implications for talar stability. Foot Ankle Int 2004;25:716–27.

51. Amanatullah DF, McDonald E, Shellito A, et al. Effect of mini-fragment fixation on the stabilization of medial malleolus fractures. J Trauma Acute Care Surg 2012;72:948–53.

52. Gorter E, Krijnen P, Schipper I. Vitamin D status and adult fracture healing. J Clin Orthop Trauma 2017; 8:34–7.

53. Eschle D, Aeschlimann A. Is supplementation of vitamin D beneficial for fracture healing? A short review of the literature. Geriatr Orthop Surg Rehabil 2011;2:90–3.

54. Doetsch A, Faber J, Lynnerup N, et al. The effect of calcium and vitamin D3 supplementation on the healing of the proximal humerus fracture: a randomized placebo-controlled study. Calcif Tissue Int 2004;75:183–8.

55. Kolb J, Schilling A, Bischoff J. Calcium homeostasis influences radiological fracture healing in postmenopausal women. Arch Orthop Trauma Surg 2013; 133:187–92.

56. Fischer V, Haffner-Luntzer M, Prystaz K, et al. Calcium and vitamin-D deficiency marginally impairs fracture healing but aggravates posttraumatic bone loss in osteoporotic mice. Sci Rep 2017;7:7223.

Surgical Considerations for Vitamin D Deficiency in Foot and Ankle Surgery

Kenneth DeFontes III, MD[a,b], Jeremy T. Smith, MD[a,*]

KEYWORDS

- Vitamin D • Deficiency • Hypovitaminosis D • Bone marrow edema syndrome (BMES)
- Foot and ankle

KEY POINTS

- A substantial percentage of patients undergoing foot and ankle surgery are vitamin D deficient.
- Consideration should be given for preoperative vitamin D testing in at-risk patients undergoing foot and ankle surgery.
- Vitamin D repletion either preoperatively or postoperatively is a proposed way to optimize outcomes in orthopedic surgery, including foot and ankle surgery.
- There may be a correlation between vitamin D deficiency and poor clinical outcomes.
- Vitamin D supplementation is relatively safe and inexpensive.

INTRODUCTION

Vitamin D deficiency is extremely common, affecting more than one billion people worldwide.[1] There are many known causes of vitamin D deficiency, including malnutrition, malabsorption syndromes, and inadequate sun exposure. Vitamin D level has been shown to correlate to both climate and geography, which is in part thought to be due to variations in sunlight, which affects vitamin D metabolism (**Fig. 1**).[2,3] Vitamin D deficiency is particularly prevalent in certain populations. For example, patients with darker skin living in areas with less sun exposure are at particular risk for low vitamin D.[1,3,4] Certain medical conditions also predispose to vitamin D deficiency, including patients with gastrointestinal malabsorption syndromes and renal insufficiency.[1]

Relating to orthopedics, certain patient subgroups have been noted to be at particular risk for low vitamin D levels. These subgroups include orthopedic trauma patients,[5–11] geriatric hip and fragility fracture patients,[12–15] patients undergoing joint replacement surgery,[16–25] spinal fusion patients,[26–28] those undergoing scoliosis correction,[29] and patients with foot and ankle conditions.[30–35] This article summarizes the current literature regarding vitamin D deficiency in patients undergoing orthopedic surgery, focusing on patients with foot and ankle conditions.

VITAMIN D METABOLISM

A general understanding of vitamin D metabolism is necessary to appreciate the intricate relationship between vitamin D levels, calcium homeostasis, and bone health (see **Fig. 1**). Vitamin D is absorbed both through the skin and through the gastrointestinal tract. Vitamin D2, also known as ergocalciferol, is derived from plant sources and generated by UV

Disclosure Statement: Dr J.T. Smith and Dr K. DeFontes have no commercial or financial conflicts of interest and have not received any funding related to the topic of this article.

a Department of Orthopaedics, Brigham and Women's Hospital, 75 Francis Street, Boston, MA 02115, USA; b Towson Orthopaedic Associates, Ruxton Professional Center, 8322 Bellona Avenue, Suite 100, Towson, MD 21204, USA

* Corresponding author. Brigham and Women's Faulkner Hospital, 1153 Centre Street, Suite 4 South, Jamaica Plain, MA 02130.

E-mail address: jsmith42@bwh.harvard.edu

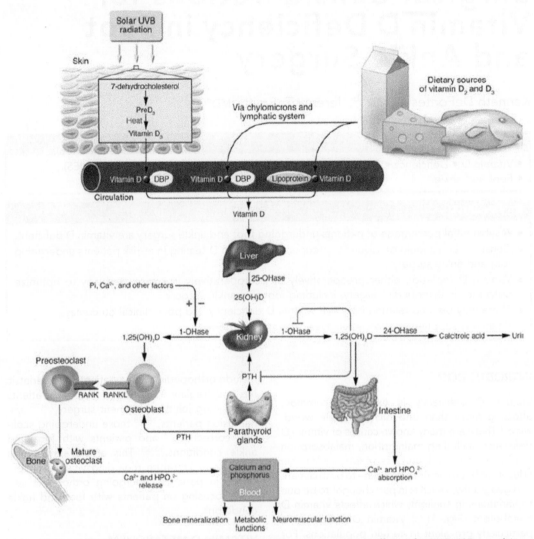

Fig. 1. Photoproduction and metabolism of vitamin D and the various biologic effects of 1,25(OH)2D on calcium, phosphorus, and bone metabolism. DBP, Vitamin D Binding Protein. (*From* McCabe MP, Smyth MP, Richardson DR. Current concept review: vitamin D and stress fractures. Foot Ankle Int 2012;33(6):527; with permission.)

radiation of ergosterol from yeast.[1] Vitamin D3 is called cholecalciferol and is generated from the UV irradiation of 7-dehydrocholesterol from lanolin, which is found in animals.[1,36] Both vitamin D2 and vitamin D3 are converted to 25-hydroxyvitamin D (25(OH)D) in the liver. This major circulating metabolite, also called calcidiol, is the most commonly measured vitamin D laboratory value.

Calcidiol (25(OH)D) circulates in the blood and undergoes hydroxylation in the kidneys to become calcitriol (1,25(OH)D).[1,36] As the active form of vitamin D, calcitriol affects both bone turnover and gastrointestinal absorption to regulate calcium and phosphate levels. In the setting of vitamin D deficiency, less calcium is

absorbed from the gastrointestinal track, which upregulates parathyroid hormone (PTH).[1,37,38] Increased PTH has the effect of increasing bone resorption, which can lead to osteoporosis, osteomalacia/rickets, and compromised bone healing.[1,39]

VITAMIN D AND MUSCULOSKELETAL HEALTH

Vitamin D levels are reported in either nanograms per milliliter or nanomoles per liter. Calcidiol (25(OH)D) is the value measured in most routine laboratory tests. Although there is no universally accepted classification of vitamin D deficiency or insufficiency, there is a consensus in the literature regarding normal values. The Endocrine Society defines vitamin D insufficiency as between 20 and 30 ng/mL and vitamin D deficiency as less than 20 ng/mL.[40] Patients with values greater than 30 ng/mL are considered sufficient (Table 1). Most of the studies in the orthopedic and foot and ankle literature use the Endocrine Society definition of vitamin D adequacy, and unless otherwise noted, all articles referenced in this chapter use this definition.

Vitamin D is critical to bone health due to its regulation of serum calcium and phosphate. In the most basic sense, low levels of vitamin D result in low levels of calcium. In one of the most striking examples of vitamin D deficiency, rickets, bone is exceptionally soft and weakened, which results in delayed growth and skeletal deformity.[1,3,39] In cases of renal osteodystrophy, effective vitamin D deficiency results in substantial bone weakness and fracture risk.[1,37] These examples illustrate the integral role that vitamin D plays in bone health. Similarly, low vitamin D has been identified as a common cause of fragility fractures in patients without known medical underlying risk factors for vitamin D deficiency.[12–14,41] Fragility fractures are not only an enormous burden to the elderly population, in which they most commonly occur, but also an economic burden to the health care system.[1,42]

In addition to the well-documented effects of vitamin D on bone homeostasis, vitamin D also directly affects muscle. Adequate vitamin D levels have been associated with minimizing risks of falls, suggesting a connection between vitamin D and muscle strength.[1,43,44] Vitamin D interacts directly with muscle through the vitamin D receptor that is found in skeletal muscle.[43,45,46] Additional research is needed to fully elucidate the role of vitamin D and skeletal muscle health and function.

For supplementation in those with adequate vitamin D levels, the Endocrine Society Clinical Practice Guidelines recommend at least 600 IU of vitamin D daily for patients age 1 to 70 and at least 800 IU daily for patients over the age of 70, with a general upper limit of 4000 IU daily for adults.[40,47] For those found to be deficient of vitamin D, it is recommended that children aged

1 to 18 take 2000 IU daily or a 6-week course of 50,000 IU weekly followed by 400 to 1000 IU daily.[40] Adults with deficiency are recommended 6000 IU daily or 50,000 IU weekly for 8 weeks followed by maintenance treatment of 1500 to 2000 IUs daily.[40] The goal of treatment is to maintain levels greater than 30 ng/mL. Either D2 or D3 supplementation is acceptable.[40]

Vitamin D toxicity has been described and is extremely rare. Levels greater than 150 ng/mL are considered excessive and can result in intoxication.[48] Symptoms of vitamin D intoxication range from mild gastrointestinal distress (nausea, vomiting, and diarrhea) to more severe symptoms, including lethargy, headache, cardiac arrhythmia, muscle and joint pain, frequent urination, and kidney stones.[48,49]

VITAMIN D IN ORTHOPEDIC TRAUMA

The rate of vitamin D deficiency is particularly high in orthopedic trauma patients, including both low-energy and high-energy trauma.[7,10,11,13,41] In the geriatric hip fracture population, vitamin D levels have been reported to be as high as 76%.[13] Nevertheless, despite high rates of deficiency among those with fractures, it is not clear that vitamin D deficiency affects outcomes after fracture. A recent meta-analysis evaluated vitamin D supplementation in fracture patients and found that vitamin D supplementation was a safe way to increase vitamin D levels in all cases, but it was not clear whether supplementation affected outcomes.[9] Similarly, a study from Singapore did not show any effect of vitamin D deficiency on clinical outcomes in 171 patients with geriatric hip fractures.[15] Lee and colleagues[13] in 2015 looked at vitamin D deficiency as a risk factor for mortality in older patients with a hip fracture and found no correlation between serum 25(OH)D levels and mortality. Although vitamin D levels may not affect clinical outcomes after trauma, some researchers think that vitamin D has an important role in fracture prevention. A large meta-analysis published in 2005 concluded that vitamin D supplementation (700–800 IU daily) reduced the risk of hip and any nonvertebral fractures in ambulatory or institutionalized elderly patients.[50]

Nonunions in trauma patients have been linked to vitamin D deficiency. In 2007, Brinker and colleagues[5] investigated 683 patients who developed a nonunion from a fracture over a 7-year period. The investigators identified patients in whom a metabolic cause for nonunion was suspected by identifying those with adequate fracture stabilization and reduction, those who had a history of multiple low-energy fractures, and those with a

Table 1		
Normal 25-hydroxyvitamin D values and cutoffs for insufficiency and deficiency		
Diagnosis	**Values (ng/mL)**	**Values (nmol/L)**
Sufficient	>30	>75
Insufficient	21–29	52.5–72.5
Deficient	<20	<50

nonunited pubic rami or sacral ala fracture. Thirty-seven patients were identified and referred to an endocrinologist. Of these, 68% were found to be vitamin D deficient. Although this study does not definitively identify a causal link between low vitamin D levels and the development of nonunion, most patients deemed to be at highest risk for nonunion had vitamin D deficiency.

The orthopedic trauma literature also sheds light on the effectiveness of vitamin D supplementation in patients with vitamin D deficiency. In 2015, Robertson and colleagues[8] monitored vitamin D levels of 201 orthopedic trauma patients throughout the course of treatment. Before initiation of vitamin D therapy, the rate of vitamin D deficiency was 40% and the rate of insufficiency was 44%. All patients, regardless of preoperative levels, received 1000 IU D3 and 1500 mg of calcium daily, and those insufficient or deficient additionally received 50,000 IU D2 weekly for 8 weeks. Vitamin D levels in all patients improved throughout follow-up, but most patients did not normalize. These data suggest that supplementation can improve vitamin D levels, although attention should be given to dosing and duration of supplementation.

VITAMIN D IN ELECTIVE ORTHOPEDIC SURGERY

Vitamin D deficiency has been reported to be present in up to 86% of patients undergoing elective orthopedic procedures.[16,18,27,28,31,51,52] Patients undergoing elective hip and knee replacement have been found to have a particularly high prevalence of vitamin D deficiency.[16,22] For comparison, although rates of vitamin D deficiency tend to vary geographically, an analysis of healthy adults aged 18 to 29 in the United States reported 36% had 25(OH)D levels less than or equal to 20 ng/mL.[53,54] A study of healthy patients in France reported a deficiency rate of 14%.[55] Although these groups vary in terms of age, many studies evaluating elective orthopedic patients report substantially higher rates of deficiency than population norms.

Studies have shown that patients with lower preoperative vitamin D levels have lower preoperative functional status.[21] Whether this is due to a causal effect of vitamin D or is representative of poorer general fitness is uncertain. Studies also suggest that patients with lower vitamin D levels have lower outcome scores after total knee and hip replacement.[23,24,56] Shin and colleagues[24] analyzed a prospective cohort of 92 patients who underwent total knee arthroplasty and found that mean postoperative Knee Society Scores and additional performance tests were significantly lower in the vitamin D deficient group. Unnanuntana and colleagues[25] showed that early postoperative functional outcomes, at 6 weeks, were similar in patients who were deficient versus sufficient preoperatively, as long as adequate vitamin D supplementation was begun as soon as it was identified. Additional research is needed to fully elucidate the effects of vitamin D deficiency and supplementation in the arthroplasty population.

There also appears to be a link between vitamin D and periprosthetic infection rate, length of hospital stay, and overall complication rates after elective orthopedic surgery.[17,19,20,22] Hegde and colleagues[17] evaluated 6598 patients undergoing elective joint replacement in the Humana registry and found those with vitamin D deficiency to have a statistically higher rate of periprosthetic surgical site infection and prosthesis explantation as well as a higher overall complication rate. Similarly, Maier and colleagues[19] found significant differences in vitamin D levels in patients who developed an infection after hip, knee, or shoulder arthroplasty when compared with patients who were either scheduled for arthroplasty or developed aseptic loosening. Maier and colleagues[20] also reported longer hospital stays in those with vitamin D deficiency in 1083 patients undergoing elective hip or knee arthroplasty.

VITAMIN D IN FOOT AND ANKLE SURGERY

Much of the early literature looking at hypovitaminosis D and foot and ankle patients relates to bone marrow edema syndrome, also known as transient osteoporosis.[57] Bone marrow edema syndrome is characterized by a sudden onset of severe periarticular pain without trauma and has a predilection for the lower extremities, including the hip, knee, foot, and ankle.[57,58] Multiple studies have evaluated the association between vitamin D and bone marrow edema syndrome in the foot and have found vitamin D deficiency in 84% to 90% of these patients.[57,59,60] Treatment of bone marrow edema syndrome is largely nonsurgical and includes off-loading, synthetic prostacyclin analogues, bisphosphonates, and vitamin D supplementation.[57] When combined with other medical therapies, such as bisphosphonates, vitamin D supplementation seems to cause some improvement in pain, suggesting vitamin D supplementation may be an important part of treatment of these patients.[59–61]

More recently, studies have examined rates of hypovitaminosis D in patients with foot and ankle injuries (Table 2). In 2014, Smith and colleagues[33] evaluated the prevalence of vitamin D deficiency in patients who presented with acute low-energy foot and ankle injuries. The study cohort included patients with a low-energy ankle fracture, fifth metatarsal base fracture, or stress fracture of the foot and ankle. A group of patients with an ankle sprain were used as a control. Of patients with a low-energy foot or ankle fracture, 47% were vitamin D insufficient, with 13% of patients severely deficient. These values were statistically significantly lower than in the control group, of which 71% had normal vitamin D levels. Further analysis revealed an association between low vitamin D and smoking, obesity, and other medical risk factors for hypovitaminosis D. This study demonstrated that vitamin D deficiency is particularly common among patients with a low-energy fracture of the foot or ankle. Although foot and

ankle injuries are not typically classified as fragility fractures, the investigators suggest that clinicians consider these injuries to be related to overall bone health. Accordingly, consideration should be given to checking vitamin D levels in patients who present with low-energy foot or ankle injuries.

Vitamin D levels have also been evaluated in elective foot and ankle surgery populations. A study published in 2017 evaluated 577 patients in England undergoing elective foot and ankle surgery.[30] This large cohort reported the levels of vitamin D to be normally distributed, yet with only 18% of patients within the normal range. The investigators noted an association between the season and vitamin D levels, which can likely be attributed to levels of sun exposure.

In 2016, Michelson and colleagues[31] looked at a series of 81 patients undergoing ankle, hindfoot, or midfoot arthrodesis. Within this cohort,

Table 2 Summary of studies evaluating foot and ankle conditions and vitamin D		
Authors	**Level of Evidence**	**Major Conclusions**
Bogunovic et al,[52] 2010	Retrospective review	Inadequate vitamin D levels were found in 34% of 192 patients who underwent foot and ankle surgery, of which 32% were deficient
Smith et al,[33] 2014	Prospective case control	Vitamin D insufficiency was found in 47% of patients with foot and ankle injuries, of which in 13% were deficient. Vitamin D values were lower in patients with a fracture compared with patients with a sprain
Michelson et al,[31] 2016	Prospective study	Hypovitaminosis D was found in 67% of 118 patients undergoing elective ankle, hindfoot, or midfoot arthrodesis
Warner et al,[35] 2016	Retrospective review of prospective patient registry	Vitamin D insufficiency was present in 32% of patients operatively treated for ankle fracture, and vitamin D deficiency was present in 37%. Patients with vitamin D deficiency had worse FAOS scores in some domains than those who with levels greater than 20 ng/mL
Aujla et al,[30] 2017	Prospective cohort	Hypovitaminosis D was present in 83% of a total of 577 patients undergoing elective foot and ankle surgery
Moore et al,[32] 2017	Retrospective case control	Hypovitaminosis D was present in 48% of patients who developed a nonunion after elective foot and ankle reconstruction compared with 10% of patients who underwent successful fusion
Telleria et al,[34] 2018	Comparative study	Hypovitaminosis D was identified in 54% of patients with an osteochondral lesion of the talus compared with 28% of patients with an ankle sprain

67% of patients were found to have low vitamin D levels (<30 ng/mL). Interestingly, older patients had a statistically lower risk for hypovitaminosis D. The investigators also looked at the Charlson Co-Morbidity Index.[62] Patients with a Charlson Co-Morbidity Index greater than or equal to 3, which corresponds to either patients with diabetes or multiple comorbid conditions, were at increased risk for vitamin D deficiency. To address the deficiency, all patients were placed on 2000 IU D3 and 750 mg calcium carbonate daily and those with hypovitaminosis D were also treated with 50,000 IU D2 three times a week for 2 to 3 months. Despite this repletion, only 56% of patients who were deficient corrected to normal levels. This study illustrates 2 important points. The prevalence of vitamin D deficiency in patients undergoing foot and ankle fusions, at least in Vermont, is quite high. Second, the repletion approach used in this study failed to adequately normalize levels in many patients.

An additional group of patients who have been recently studied are those with osteochondral lesions of the talus (OLTs). Patients with OLTs have a particularly high rate of vitamin D deficiency, as identified by Telleria and colleagues.[34] In patients with a documented OLT, the prevalence of vitamin D insufficiency is 54%. This rate of hypovitaminosis contrasts with an acute ankle sprain. These data suggest that OLTs may be related to an underlying bone abnormality, and the investigators suggest that patients presenting with a talar osteochondral lesion should be evaluated for vitamin D sufficiency. Although repletion was not evaluated in this study, the implication is that vitamin D and overall bone health should be considered when treating patients with OLT. Other studies have looked at juvenile osteochondritis dissecans and have similarly found high rates of vitamin D deficiency, ranging from 60% to 78%.[63,64]

The relationship between vitamin D deficiency and nonunion has also been studied in patients undergoing foot and ankle surgery.[32] Twenty-nine patients who underwent successful arthrodesis (forefoot, midfoot, hindfoot, ankle) were matched to 29 patients who developed a nonunion after an arthrodesis procedure. Vitamin D deficiency or insufficiency was identified in 48% of patients who developed a nonunion, compared with 10% in patients who united. Statistical analysis revealed that patients with a preoperative diagnosis of vitamin D insufficiency or deficiency were 8 times more likely to develop a nonunion than patients who had sufficient vitamin

D levels. Although this study is small and cannot definitively link hypovitaminosis D and nonunion, these data suggest that an association may exist between vitamin D and the development of nonunion in foot and ankle surgery. Further study into these relationships is needed.

With respect to treatment of hypovitaminosis D, there are very few studies that examine the benefits of treatment on outcomes after foot and ankle surgery. In a study examining hypovitaminosis D in patients undergoing ankle fracture fixation, Warner and colleagues[35] reported improved outcomes in patients who were vitamin D sufficient. In this study, the investigators identified a hypovitaminosis D prevalence of 69% in a registry of 98 patients. Patients with vitamin D deficiency had statistically lower Foot and Ankle Outcome Score (FAOS), specifically in the symptoms and quality-of-life domains. Whether the poorer outcome was due to the vitamin D level or if this was an indication of poorer overall fitness is not known. If an association between vitamin D and outcomes does exist, one can theorize as to why vitamin D is beneficial. This benefit could be due to direct effects on bone healing or alternatively influencing balance and muscle strength and thus facilitating better rehabilitation and recovery.[43,65,66]

With respect to postoperative rehabilitation after foot and ankle surgery, vitamin D has been shown to benefit skeletal muscle and athletic performance. A recent review examines the role of vitamin D in muscle function.[43] Skeletal muscle has a vitamin D receptor that, once activated, enhances the interaction between myosin and actin. In a murine knockout model, mice without functional vitamin D receptors have been shown to have smaller muscle fiber size and body weight compared with normal mice, even when calcium levels are normalized.[43,67] Vitamin D is thus postulated to have a direct effect on muscle strength, performance, and recovery.[43,45] Additional research is necessary to further develop the understanding of the complex interplay between vitamin D and muscle strength, particularly as it pertains to recovery after injury or surgery.

SUMMARY

In summary, vitamin D deficiency is common in patients undergoing orthopedic procedures, including patients with foot and ankle conditions and those undergoing foot and ankle surgery. As the understanding and awareness of vitamin D and bone health evolve, we continue to identify conditions in which vitamin D deficiency is clinically relevant. The limited data available to date suggest that patients who are vitamin D sufficient may have improved outcomes. The authors would thus recommend monitoring vitamin D levels as part of the preoperative evaluation for certain foot and ankle conditions. Because of its low cost and ease of administration, vitamin D optimization should be a routine consideration before orthopedic surgery.

REFERENCES

1. Holick MF. Vitamin D deficiency. N Engl J Med 2007;357:266–81.

2. Holick MF, Chen TC, Lu Z, et al. Vitamin D and skin physiology a D-lightful story. J Bone Miner Res 2007;22:V28–33.

3. Pettifor JM, Moodley GP, Hough FS, et al. The effect of season and latitude on in vitro vitamin D formation by sunlight in South Africa. S Afr Med J 1996;86:1270–2.

4. Vieth R. Why the optimal requirements for vitamin D3 is probably much higher than what is officially recommended for adults. J Steroid Biochem Mol Biol 2004;89-90:575–9.

5. Brinker MR, O'Conner DP, Monla YT, et al. Metabolic and endocrine abnormalities in patients with nonunions. J Orthop Trauma 2007;21:557–70.

6. Feng Y, Cheng G, Wang H, et al. The associations between serum 25-hydroxyvitamin D level and the risk of total fracture and hip fracture. Osteoporos Int 2017;28:1641–52.

7. Hood MA, Murtha YM, Della Rocca GJ, et al. Prevalence of low vitamin D levels in patients with orthopaedic trauma. Am J Orthop 2016;45:E522–6.

8. Robertson DS, Jenkins T, Murtha YM, et al. Effectiveness of vitamin D therapy in orthopaedic trauma patients. J Orthop Trauma 2015;29:e451–3.

9. Sprague S, Petrisor B, Scott T, et al. What is the role of vitamin D supplementation in acute fracture patients? A systematic review and meta-analysis of the prevalence of hypovitaminosis D and supplementation efficacy. J Orthop Trauma 2016;30:53–63.

10. Steele B, Serota A, Helfet DL, et al. Vitamin D deficiency: a common occurrence in both high- and low-energy fractures. HSS J 2008;4:143–8.

11. Zellner BS, Dawson JR, Reichel LM, et al. Prospective nutritional analysis of a diverse trauma population demonstrates substantial hypovitaminosis D. J Orthop Trauma 2014;28:e210–5.

12. Buchebner D, McGuigan F, Gerdhem P, et al. Association between hypovitaminosis D in elderly women and long- and short-term mortality – results from the Osteoporotic Prospective Risk Assessment Cohort. J Am Geriatr Soc 2016;64:990–7.

13. Lee GH, Lim JW, Park YG, et al. Vitamin D deficiency is highly concomitant but not strong risk factor for mortality in patients aged 50 years and older with hip fracture. J Bone Metab 2015;22:205–9.

14. Maier GS, Seeger JB, Horas K, et al. The prevalence of vitamin D deficiency in patients with vertebral fragility fractures. Bone Joint J 2015;97-B:89–93.

15. Seng WR, Belani MH, Ramason R, et al. Functional improvement in geriatric hip fractures: does vitamin D deficiency affect the functional outcome of patients with surgically treated interochanteric hip fractures. Geriatr Orthop Surg Rehabil 2015;6:186–91.

16. Glowacki J, Hurwitz S, Thornhill TS, et al. Osteoporosis and vitamin-D deficiency among postmenopausal women with osteoarthritis undergoing total hip arthroplasty. J Bone Joint Surg Am 2003;85-A:2371–7.

17. Hegde V, Arshi A, Wang C, et al. Preoperative vitamin D deficiency is associated with higher postoperative complication rates in total knee arthroplasty. Orthopedics 2018;27:1–7.

18. Inkrott BP, Koberling JL, Noel CR. Hypovitaminosis D in patients undergoing shoulder arthroplasty: a single-center analysis. Orthopedics 2016;39:e651–6.

19. Maier GS, Hora K, Seeger JB, et al. Is there an association between periprosthetic joint infection and low vitamin D levels? Int Orthop 2014;38:1499–504.

20. Maier GS, Maus U, Lazovic D, et al. Is there an association between low serum 25-OH-D levels and the length of hospital stay in orthopaedic patients after arthroplasty? J Orthop Traumatol 2016;17:297–302.

21. Maniar RN, Patil AM, Maniar AR, et al. Effect of preoperative vitamin D levels on functional performance after total knee arthroplasty. Clin Orthop Surg 2016;8:153–6.

22. Russell LA. Osteoporosis and orthopedic surgery: effect of bone health on total joint arthroplasty outcome. Curr Rheumatol Rep 2013;15:371.

23. Schwartz FH, Lange J. Factors that affect outcome following total joint arthroplasty: a review of the recent literature. Curr Rev Musculoskelet Med 2017;10:346–55.

24. Shin KY, Park KK, Moon SH, et al. Vitamin D deficiency adversely affects early post-operative functional outcomes after total knee arthroplasty. Knee Surg Sports Traumatol Arthrosc 2017;25:3424–30.

25. Unnanuntana A, Saleh A, Nguyen JT, et al. Low vitamin D status does not adversely affect short-term functional outcome after total hip arthroplasty. J Arthroplasty 2013;28:315–22.

26. Kim TH, Yoon JY, Lee BH, et al. Changes in vitamin D status after surgery in female patients with lumbar spinal stenosis and its clinical significance. Spine 2012;37:E1326–30.

27. Mabey T, Singhatanadgige W, Yingsakmongkol W, et al. Vitamin D and spine surgery. World J Orthop 2016;18:726–30.

28. Stoker GE, Buchowski JM, Bridwell KH, et al. Pre-operative vitamin D status of adults undergoing surgical spinal fusion. Spine 2013;15:507–15.

29. Mayes T, Anadio JM, Sturm PF. Prevalence of vitamin D deficiency in pediatric patients with scoliosis preparing for spinal surgery. Spine Deform 2017;5:369–73.

30. Aujla RS, Allen PE, Ribbans WJ. Vitamin D levels in 577 consecutive elective foot & ankle surgery patients. Foot Ankle Surg 2017 [pii:S1268-7731(17)31368-1].

31. Michelson JD, Charlson MD. Vitamin D status in an elective orthopaedic surgical population. Foot Ankle Int 2016;37:186–91.

32. Moore KR, Howell MA, Saltrick KR, et al. Risk factors associated with nonunion after elective foot and ankle reconstruction: a case-control study. Foot Ankle Surg 2017;56:457–62.

33. Smith JT, Halim K, Palms DA, et al. Prevalence of vitamin D deficiency in patients with foot and ankle injuries. Foot Ankle Int 2014;35:8–13.

34. Telleria JS, Ready LV, Bluman EB, et al. Prevalence of vitamin D deficiency in patients with talar osteochondral lesions. Foot Ankle Int 2018;39:471–8.

35. Warner SJ, Garner MR, Nguyen JT, et al. Perioperative vitamin D levels correlate with clinical outcomes after ankle fracture fixation. Arch Orthop Trauma Surg 2016;136:339–44.

36. Christakos S, Dhawan P, Verstuyf A, et al. Vitamin D: metabolism, molecular mechanisms of action, and pleiotrophic effects. Physiol Rev 2016;96:365–408.

37. Holick MF. Vitamin D for health in chronic kidney disease. Semin Dial 2005;18:266–75.

38. Thomas KK, Lloyd-Jones DM, Thadhani RI, et al. Hypovitaminosis D in medical inpatients. N Engl J Med 1998;338:777–83.

39. Holick MF. Ressurection of vitamin D deficiency and rickets. J Clin Invest 2006;116:2062–72.

40. Holick MF, Binkley NC, Bischoff-Ferarri HA, et al. Evaluation, treatment, and prevention of vitamin D deficiency: an Endocrine Society clinical practice guideline. J Clin Endocrinol Metab 2011;96:1911–30.

41. Leboff MS, Kohlmeier L, Hurwitz S, et al. Occult vitamin D deficiency in postmenopausal US women with acute hip fracture. JAMA 1999;281:1505–11.

42. Orsini LS, Rousculp MD, Long SR, et al. Healthcare utilization and expenditures in the United States: a study of osteoporosis-related fractures. Osteoporos Int 2005;16:359–71.

43. Abrams GD, Feldman D, Safran MR. Effects of vitamin D on skeletal muscle and athletic performance. J Am Acad Orthop Surg 2018;26:278–85.

44. Bischoff-Ferrari HA, Giovannucci E, Willett WC, et al. Estimation of optimal serum concentrations of 25-hydroxyvitamin D for multiple health outcomes. Am J Clin Nutr 2006;84:18–28.

45. Costa EM, Blau HM, Feldman D. 1,25-dihydroxyvitamin D3 receptors and hormonal responses in cloned human skeletal muscle cells. Endocrinology 1986;199:2214–20.

46. Pojednic RM, Ceglia L. The emerging biomolecular role of vitamin D in skeletal muscle. Exerc Sport Sci Rev 2014;42:76–81.

47. Ross AC, Manson JE, Abrams SA, et al. The 2011 report on dietary reference intakes for calcium and vitamin D from the Institute of Medicine: what clinicians need to know. J Clin Endocrinol Metab 2011;96:53–8.

48. Alshahrani F, Aljohani N. Vitamin D: deficiency, sufficiency, and toxicity. Nutrients 2013;5:4605–16.

49. Schwalfenberg G. Not enough vitamin D: health consequences for Canadians. Can Fam Physician 2007;53:841–54.

50. Bischoff-Ferrari HA, Willet WC, Wong JB, et al. Fracture prevention with vitamin D supplementation: a meta-analysis of randomized controlled trials. JAMA 2005;293:2257–64.

51. Nawabi DH, Chin KF, Keen RW, et al. Vitamin D deficiency in patients with osteoarthritis undergoing total hip replacement: a cause for concern? J Bone Joint Surg Br 2010;92:496–9.

52. Bogunovic L, Kim AD, Beamer BS, et al. Hypovitaminosis D in patients scheduled to undergo orthopaedic surgery: a single-center analysis. J Bone Joint Surg Am 2010;92:2300–4.

53. Holick MF. High prevalence of vitamin D inadequacy and implications for health. Mayo Clin Proc 2008;81:353–73.

54. Tangpricha V, Pearce EN, Chen TC, et al. Vitamin D insufficiency among free-living healthy young adults. Am J Med 2002;112:659–62.

55. Chapuy MC, Preziosi P, Maamer M, et al. Prevalence of vitamin D insufficiency in an adult normal population. Osteoporos Int 1997;7:439–43.

56. Lavernia CJ, Villa JM, Iacobelli DA, et al. Vitamin D insufficiency in patients with THA: prevalence and effects on outcome. Clin Orthop Relat Res 2014;472:681–6.

57. Mirghasemi SA, Trepman E, Sadeghi MS. Bone marrow edema syndrome in the foot and ankle. Foot Ankle Int 2016;37:1364–73.

58. Gigena LM, Chung CB, Lektrakul N, et al. Transient bone marrow edema of the talus: MR imaging findings in five patients. Skeletal Radiol 2002;31:202–7.

59. Sprinchorn AE, O'Sullivan R, Beischer AD. Transient bone marrow edema of the foot and ankle and its association with reduced systemic bone mineral density. Foot Ankle Int 2011;32:508–12.

60. Horas K, Fraissler L, Maier G, et al. High prevalence of vitamin D deficiency in patients with bone marrow edema syndrome of the foot and ankle. Foot Ankle Int 2017;38:760–6.

61. Ringe JD, Dorst A, Faber H. Effective and rapid treatment of painful localized transient

osteoporosis (bone marrow edema) with intravenous ibandronate. Osteoporos Int 2005;16:2063–8.

62. Charlson ME, Pompei P, Ales KL, et al. A new method of classifying prognostic comorbidity in longitudinal studies: development and validation. J Chronic Dis 1987;40:373–83.

63. Bruns J, Werner M, Soyka M. Is vitamin D insufficiency or deficiency related to the development of osteochondritis dissecans? Knee Surg Sports Traumatol Arthrosc 2016;24:1575–9.

64. Maier GS, Lazovic D, Maus U, et al. Vitamin D deficiency: the missing etiological factors in the development of juvenile osteochondrosis dissecans? J Pediatr Orthop 2016. [Epub ahead of print].

65. Houston DK, Cesari M, Ferruci L, et al. Association between vitamin D status and physical performance: the InCHANTI study. J Gerontol A Biol Sci Med Sci 2007;62:440–6.

66. Tomlinson PB, Joseph C, Angioni M. Effects of vitamin D supplementation on upper and lower body muscle strength levels in healthy individuals: a systematic review with meta-analysis. J Sci Med Sport 2015;18:575–80.

67. Endo I, Inoue D, Mitsui T, et al. Deletion of vitamin D receptor gene in mice results in abnormal skeletal muscle development with deregulated expression of myoregulatory transcription factors. Endocrinology 2003;144:5138–44.

Moving?

Make sure your subscription moves with you!

To notify us of your new address, find your **Clinics Account Number** (located on your mailing label above your name), and contact customer service at:

Email: journalscustomerservice-usa@elsevier.com

800-654-2452 (subscribers in the U.S. & Canada)
314-447-8871 (subscribers outside of the U.S. & Canada)

Fax number: 314-447-8029

Elsevier Health Sciences Division
Subscription Customer Service
3251 Riverport Lane
Maryland Heights, MO 63043

*To ensure uninterrupted delivery of your subscription, please notify us at least 4 weeks in advance of move.

Moving?

Make sure your subscription moves with you!

To notify us of your new address, find your Clinics Account Number (located on your mailing label above your name), and contact customer service at:

Email: journalscustomerservice-usa@elsevier.com

800-654-2452 (subscribers in the U.S. & Canada)
314-447-8871 (subscribers outside of the U.S. & Canada)

Fax number: 314-447-8029

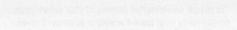

Elsevier Health Sciences Division
Subscription Customer Service
3251 Riverport Lane
Maryland Heights, MO 63043

Printed and bound by CPI Group (UK) Ltd, Croydon, CR0 4YY

08/05/2025

01864741-0008